THE SOUTH BEACH DIET GOOD FATS GOOD CARBS GUIDE

Dr ARTHUR AGATSTON

**Author of *The South Beach Diet*,
the Revolutionary International Bestseller**

RODALE

This edition first published in the UK in 2004 by
Rodale Ltd
7–10 Chandos Street
London W1G 9AD
www.rodale.co.uk

Printed and bound in the UK by CPI Bath using acid-free paper from
sustainable sources.

1 3 5 7 9 8 6 4 2

Book design by Carol Angstadt

A CIP record for this book is available from the British Library
ISBN: 1–4050–6715–2

This paperback edition distributed to the book trade by Pan Macmillan Ltd

Notice
This book is intended as a reference volume only, not as a medical manual. The information given here is designed to help you make informed decisions about your health.
It is not intended as a substitute for any treatment that may have been prescribed by your
doctor. If you suspect that you have a medical problem, we urge you to seek competent
medical help.

Mention of specific companies, organizations or authorities in this book does not
imply endorsement by the publisher, nor does mention of specific companies, organizations or authorities imply that they endorse this book.

Internet addresses and telephone numbers given in this book were accurate at the
time it went to press.

This edition has been adapted from the original US edition. Some foods that are
uncommon outside the US have been replaced with everyday items from other parts of
the world.

Portion sizes reflect those recommended on nutrition information labels in the UK.

All spoon measurements are level: 1 teaspoon = 5 ml; 1 tablespoon = 15 ml

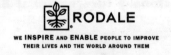

RODALE

WE **INSPIRE** AND **ENABLE** PEOPLE TO IMPROVE
THEIR LIVES AND THE WORLD AROUND THEM

CONTENTS

YOUR ROAD MAP TO SOUTH BEACH SUCCESS

Welcome! I'm glad you've decided to try the South Beach Diet and have taken the first step towards a future filled with health and vitality.

The South Beach Diet can't be classified as a low-carb diet, a low-fat diet, or a high-protein diet. Its rules: consume the right carbs and the right fats and learn to snack strategically. The South Beach Diet has been so widely successful because people lose weight without experiencing cravings or feeling deprived, or even feeling that they're *on* a diet. It allows you to enjoy 'healthy' carbohydrates, rather than the kinds that contribute to weight gain, diabetes and cardiovascular disease. You can eat a great variety of foods in a great variety of recipes. This prevents repetition and boredom, two obstacles to long-term success. Our goal is that the South

Beach Diet becomes a healthy lifestyle, not just a diet. The purpose of this Guide is to help you to accomplish this with ease. Read on for more on the principles of the diet, how to use this Guide, and shopping and eating-out tips.

Good Fats, Bad Fats

Fat is an important part of a healthy diet. There's more and more evidence that many fats are good for us and actually reduce the risk of heart attack and stroke. They also help our sugar and insulin metabolism and therefore contribute to our goals of long-term weight loss and weight maintenance. And because good fats make foods taste better, they help us enjoy the journey to a healthier lifestyle. But not all fats are created equal – there are good fats and bad fats.

'Good' fats include monounsaturated fats, found in olive and rapeseed (canola) oils, peanuts and other nuts, peanut butter and avocados. Monounsaturated fats lower total and 'bad' LDL cholesterol – which accumulates in and clogs artery walls – while maintaining levels of 'good' HDL cholesterol, which carries cholesterol from artery walls and delivers it to the liver for disposal.

Omega-3 fatty acids – polyunsaturated fats found in cold-water (oily) fish, rapeseed (canola) oil, flaxseeds (linseeds), walnuts, almonds and macadamia nuts – also count as good fat. Recent studies have shown that populations that eat more omega-3s, like Eskimos (whose diets are high in fish), have fewer serious health problems like heart disease and diabetes.

There is evidence that omega-3 oils help prevent or treat depression, arthritis and asthma and help prevent cardio-vascular disease. You'll eat both monounsaturated fats and omega-3s in abundance in all three phases of the Diet.

'Bad fats' include saturated fats – the artery-clogging kind found in butter, fatty red meats and full-fat dairy products.

'Very bad fats' are the man-made trans fats. Trans fats are created during hydrogenation, a process that turns liquid oil into solid fat, extending its shelf life. Hydrogenated oils and fats are found in many processed foods, including margarine and other spreads, ready-made pastry, biscuits, cakes and crisps (chips). Trans fats are worse than saturated fats: they are bad for our blood vessels, nervous systems and waistlines.

Hydrogenated vegetable oil must be declared in the ingre-dients' list, although trans fats don't have to be mentioned unless a specific claim has been made, such as 'low in trans fats'. (The natural trans fats in meat and milk, which act very differently in the body from the man-made kind, do not require labelling.) Here are a few ways to reduce your intake of trans fats and saturated fats, South Beach style.

Go natural: limit margarine, processed foods and fast food, which often contain high amounts of saturated and trans fats. Change your cooking methods: bake, grill, barbecue or microwave rather than fry. Remove the skin from chicken or turkey before you eat it. Cook with rapeseed (canola) or olive oil instead of butter, margarine or lard. Switch from whole milk to skimmed or semi-skimmed (low-fat) milk.

The Trans-Fat Hot List

You've probably heard a lot in the news lately about trans fats – a particularly nasty type of fat that can wreak havoc on your health. Food manufacturers have so far not been required to list this type of fat on their food labels, so here is what you need to know to identify trans fats present in foods.

Look for the words 'hydrogenated' or 'partially hydrogenated' oil or fat in the list of ingredients. If it is listed as the first, second or third ingredient, the food has a lot of trans fats in it. The common names for trans fats to look for on food labels include hydrogenated (or partially hydrogenated) vegetable oil, hydrogenated coconut oil, hydrogenated corn oil, hydrogenated soya bean oil, hydrogenated palm oil and hydrogenated vegetable oil shortening.

You can also refer to this 'Hot List' of foods that are known to contain trans fats. To keep your weight loss on track, and to maintain good health, it's best to avoid these foods as much as possible. There are plenty of great-tasting, healthier alternatives you can have instead – just check the food charts in this book!

BREADS AND BREAD PRODUCTS

Bread mixes

Bread and rolls made from chilled dough

Breadcrumb coatings

Stuffing mixes

Taco shells

White and wheat flour breads (some types)

BAKED GOODS

Most commercial bakery items, such as:

- Biscuits
- Buns
- Cakes
- Croissants

Danish pastries

Doughnuts

Muffins

Pies, pasties, quiches

Scones

DESSERTS

Most commercially prepared items, including:

- Cake decorations, sprinkles and chocolate chips
- Cakes and cake mixes
- Dessert toppings (some types)
- Fat-free cakes
- Ice cream cakes

Instant dessert mix

Pancake mix

Pie fillings (some types)

Ready-made pastry

Ready-made puddings

Ready-to-spread icing

Tart shells (pastry and biscuit crumb)

FAST FOOD

Most deep-fried fast foods and takeaway foods, including:

- Breakfast muffins
- Chicken nuggets

Fish sandwiches

French fries

Fried chicken

Fruit pies

(continued)

FATS AND OILS

Light spreads (some types)

Margarine: block and tub types

Solid vegetable fats

FROZEN FOODS

Breaded fish fingers

Chicken in sauce (some types)

Chips/French fries (some types)

Fish in sauce (some types)

Fruit pies and pie crusts

Pancakes

Pastries, tarts and pies

Pizza and pizza bases

Ready meals (some types)

Waffles

MILK AND MILK PRODUCTS

Cream alternatives (some types)

Instant cappuccino drinks

Non-dairy creamers/coffee whitener powder (some types)

Instant chocolate drinks (some types)

SALADS AND SALAD DRESSINGS

Commercially prepared salad dressings (some types)

Ready-made salads (some types)

SNACKS AND DIPS

Bean dips (some types)

Bombay mix

Cheese and cracker snack kits (some types)

Cheese dips and spreads

Cheese puffs

Chocolate- or yogurt-covered snacks (most types)

Corn chips

Crisps (chips in Australia, US)

Crackers and biscuits (some types)

Popcorn (microwave-type)

Potato puffs and sticks

Powdered dip mix

Prawn crackers

Pretzels (some types)

Tortilla chips (some types)

Weight-loss snack bars (some types)

SOUPS AND SAVOURY ITEMS

Gravy granules

Instant noodles (some types)

Packet soup

Sausage rolls

Stock cubes and granules (some types)

Vegetarian sausages (some types)

SWEETS

Most commercial confectionery, including:

Caramels

Cereal bars (some types)

Chocolate-covered sweets, nuts and raisins

Fruit chews

Yogurt-covered nuts and fruit

Good Carbs, Bad Carbs

Carbohydrates – foods that contain simple sugars (short chains of sugar molecules) or starches (long chains of sugar molecules) – have often been blamed for our epidemic of obesity and diabetes. This is only partially true, because there are both good and bad carbohydrates.

The good carbs contain important vitamins, minerals and other nutrients that are essential to our health and that help prevent heart disease and cancer. The good carbs are the ones humans were designed to consume – the unrefined ones that have contributed to our health since we began eating! Unrefined carbohydrates are found in whole, unprocessed, natural foods, such as whole grains, rice, pulses and starchy vegetables. They're also called complex carbohydrates, so named for their molecular structure. Besides being packed with fibre, vitamins and minerals, good carbs take longer to digest – a good thing, as you'll soon see.

The bad carbs, which have been consumed in unprecedented quantities in recent years (largely in an attempt to avoid fats), are the ones that have resulted in the current epidemic of obesity. Bad carbs are refined carbs, the ones where digestion has begun in factories instead of in our stomachs. Refined carbohydrates are found in processed foods, such as shop-bought baked goods, pasta and white bread.

Refined carbohydrates are often made with white flour and contain little or no fibre. White and brown flour lose nutrients along with the bran when the wheat is milled. In certain countries, including the UK and Australia, these nutrients must, by law, be replaced – usually in amounts greater than would naturally be present; this is called fortification. Current evidence suggests that fortification does not recreate the benefits of the natural vitamins that have been removed. Wholemeal flour, especially stoneground, retains all its nutrients and fibre.

Despite the fact that good carbs are a critical part of a healthy diet, the typical Western diet is filled with the bad kinds. And when we're overweight as a result of a diet laden with bad carbs, our bodies' ability to process *all* carbohydrates goes awry. To understand why, you need to understand the role of the hormone insulin.

Insulin, Fat and 'Fast Sugar'

Many foods, including natural foods like fruit and vegetables, contain naturally occurring sugar in some form, and all types of carbohydrates – both sugars and starches – are broken down during digestion into a simple sugar, glucose, that can be absorbed into the bloodstream. But there's a critical difference among these sugars: the body digests and absorbs them at different speeds.

When sugars from food enter the bloodstream, the pancreas produces insulin. It is insulin's job to move sugars out of the blood and into the cells, where they're either used or

(continued on page 16)

Beyond Weight Loss: The South Beach Diet Benefits Your Health, Too

Has your doctor told you that you must lose weight to stave off heart disease or diabetes? Then the South Beach Diet may be the one for you.

Why? Because the Diet that's helping millions shed their excess weight *didn't start out as a weight-loss diet at all*. I created the Diet to help my patients lower their levels of harmful cholesterol and triglycerides and to lower their risk of pre-diabetes (the condition that precedes full-blown type 2 diabetes and that has been linked to risk of heart attack and stroke).

And it's been proven to do just that.

To give just one example, one of my male patients in his mid-fifties had high blood pressure, high cholesterol, high triglycerides, and narrowing of his coronary arteries. His previous doctor had prescribed the usual medications. But once on the South Beach Diet, his cardiac profile quickly improved. His total cholesterol fell to a normal level – after just a month. He also lost 13.5 kg (2 st), which he's kept off, and no longer takes all those heart medications.

The results of the Diet have also been measured in a scientific setting. My colleagues and I conducted a study pitting the Diet against the strict American Heart Association diet. They randomized 40 overweight volunteers to either of the diets, meaning that half went on the Heart Association programme and half got the South Beach Diet. None of the subjects knew where their diet had come from.

After 12 weeks, five patients on the Heart Association diet had given up, compared with one on the South Beach plan. The South Beach patients also showed a greater decrease in waist-to-hip ratio, suggesting a true decrease in cardiac risk. Triglycerides dramatically decreased for the South Beach dieters, and their good-to-bad cholesterol ratio improved more than that of the Heart Association group. Finally, the South Beach dieters experienced a mean weight loss of 6.2 kg (13.6 lb), almost double the 3.4 kg (7.5 lb) lost by the Heart Association group.

stored for future use. Insulin is the key that 'unlocks' our cells and lets sugars in.

How much insulin is required to do that job depends on the foods we eat. Foods that are broken down and absorbed into the bloodstream quickly require a lot of insulin. Those that are metabolized and enter the blood more slowly require a gradual release of insulin.

In a nutshell, the quicker sugar floods the bloodstream, the quicker insulin rises. This is bad, both for your weight and for your general health.

Here's why: when glucose is absorbed slowly, the rise in blood sugar is gradual – and so is its fall, once insulin begins to work. A slow decline in blood sugar means fewer cravings later. But when blood sugar rises quickly, the pancreas pumps out a correspondingly high level of insulin. The result? Blood sugar drops so low that it triggers new cravings. Often, we satisfy cravings by overeating (typically bad carbs like chips or chocolate, cakes or biscuits), which leads to weight gain. Worse, the excess weight caused by overeating can lead to insulin resistance, the precursor to full-blown type 2 diabetes. In insulin resistance, cells ignore insulin's signal to accept glucose from the blood. As a result, the pancreas must crank out huge amounts of insulin until eventually the exhausted organ wears out.

Those of us who have grown protruding bellies while our arms and legs stay relatively thin are likely to have the syndrome of insulin resistance or 'pre-diabetes'. This occurs commonly in people with a family history of diabetes. Another sign of this syndrome is the occurrence of fatigue, weakness, headaches, irritability, shakiness, and cravings in the late morning or late afternoon. These are signs of exaggerated falls in blood sugar levels. The consumption of refined carbohydrates has unmasked this syndrome in the great majority of those of us who are overweight.

While eating the South Beach way will result in weight loss, it will also correct the way your body reacts to the very foods that made you heavy. It increases your body's sensitivity to insulin, thereby decreasing the swings in blood sugar that cause us to be hungry again, too soon after we finish a meal.

This metabolic transformation occurs in three phases. The purpose of Phase 1 is to eradicate your cravings. You will accomplish this by eliminating all starches, including all breads, potatoes and rice. You will also eliminate all sugars, including all fruits and alcoholic beverages. You will enjoy strategic snacking, eating healthy snacks like nuts or low-fat cheese before your blood sugar dips too low in the late morning, afternoon and/or evening. It takes far fewer calories to prevent those afternoon cravings than it does to satisfy those cravings once they hit. In Phase 1, nutrient-rich vegetables and healthy salads are encouraged. You can expect to lose between 3 and 6 kg (7 and 13 lb) during Phase 1.

In Phase 2, you'll gradually add back good carbohydrates, such as whole fruits and whole grains. Here's the principle for adding more carbs back: do it gradually and attentively. The goal is to eat more carbs again while continuing to lose weight. If you add an apple and a slice of bread a day and you're still losing weight, that's great. If you are having an apple, two slices of bread and a banana daily and notice that your weight loss has stalled, you've gone too far. It's time to cut back, or try some different carbs and monitor the results. You can enjoy a glass of red or white wine with a meal; drinking wine with a meal actually helps slow digestion. In this phase, weight loss is about ½ to 1 kg (1 to 2 lb) a week. You learn which carbs you can enjoy without the return of cravings.

Once you have reached your weight loss goal, it is time for Phase 3, the maintenance phase. There are no absolute restrictions here, but you have learned the 'pecking order' of the important food groups. You have learned to choose brown rice instead of white rice, sweet potatoes instead of white potatoes, and multigrain bread rather than white bread. This is where the South Beach Diet becomes a lifestyle. (For an idea of which foods to avoid and which foods to enjoy on the South Beach Diet, see the lists on the next pages.)

In the next section, you'll be introduced to a system that can help you limit foods that cause unhealthy, fat-producing spikes and dips in blood sugar and insulin and choose those that keep blood sugar steady, making it easier to lose weight and keep it off.

Introducing the Glycaemic Index

The glycaemic index (GI) is a system that ranks foods by how fast and how high they cause blood sugar to rise after eating a particular food. The GI of any particular food is always compared to a standard reference food, which is either one slice of white bread or a small amount of glucose, both of which have a numerical value of 100. The higher the glycaemic index, the greater the swings in blood sugar produced. So, in general, the lower the glycaemic index, the better the food choice. For mixed meals, the total glycaemic index is approximately the average of the indices of the individual foods.

Generally speaking, you can think of GI in three ranges: 'low' (55 and below), 'medium' (56 to 69) and 'high' (70 or above). Foods with a low GI are converted to glucose more slowly, and so their sugars enter the bloodstream more slowly. Foods with a medium or high GI, which are converted to glucose more quickly, release their sugars into the bloodstream more rapidly. This results in a swifter rise in insulin. In Australia, some foods are already labelled with their GI value.

Unrefined carbs often fall lower on the GI scale because they're rich in fibre, which takes longer to digest and so results in a slow, gradual rise in blood sugar.

(continued on page 26)

Phase 1

The following is a list of foods that you can feel free to enjoy (as well as foods you'll need to avoid) when you begin Phase 1 of the South Beach Diet. These lists will help you stay on track and avoid carbohydrates that may crop up in foods where you don't expect them.

Foods to Enjoy

SEAFOOD
All types of fish and shellfish

BEEF
Lean cuts, such as:
Sirloin (including mince)
Fillet
Topside

PORK, HAM AND BACON
Boiled ham
Lean back bacon
Pork tenderloin/fillet

POULTRY (SKINLESS)
Chicken and turkey breast
Guinea fowl
Poussin

VEAL
Chops, cutlets (trimmed of fat)
Escalope

GAME
Rabbit and hare
Venison

COLD MEATS
Fat-free or low-fat only

EGGS
Eggs are not limited unless otherwise directed by your doctor. Use egg substitute if desired.

DAIRY

Skimmed milk

Low-fat unsweetened soya milk (5 g of fat or less per serving)

Fat-free natural yogurt

Buttermilk (1% fat or less)

CHEESE (6 g of fat or less per serving)

Cheddar, reduced-fat

Cottage cheese (2% fat or less)

Dairy-free/soya cream cheese substitute

Feta

Light (low-fat) cream cheese

Mozzarella

Parmesan

Ricotta

String cheese

FATS

Oils: olive, rapeseed/canola, groundnut/peanut, walnut

Trans-fat-free butter substitute

NUTS

Almonds, 15

Brazil nuts, 8

Cashews, 15

Hazelnuts, 15

Macadamias, 8

Peanut butter, 2 tbsps

Peanuts, 20 small

Pecan or walnut halves, 15

Pine nuts, 30

Pistachios, 30

TOFU

Use natural (not deep-fried) varieties

VEGETABLES AND PULSES

Alfalfa sprouts

Artichokes (globe)

Asparagus

Aubergine/eggplant

Avocado

Beans (fresh or dried)

Beansprouts

Broccoli

Cabbage

Cauliflower

Celery

Chickpeas

Courgettes/zucchini

Cucumber

Lentils

Lettuce (all varieties)

(continued)

Foods to Enjoy (cont.)

Mangetouts (snow peas)
Mushrooms (all varieties)
Onions
Peppers
Spinach
Split peas
Spring onions
Swiss chard
Tomatoes
Turnips
Water chestnuts
Watercress

SPICES AND SEASONINGS
Herbs
Spices
Stock
Extracts (almond, vanilla, etc)
Garlic

Ginger
Hot-pepper sauce
Lemon and lime juice
Marmite, Vegemite
Mustard
Pepper (black, cayenne, paprika, white)
Soy sauce, light
Vinegar
Worcestershire sauce

**SWEET TREATS
(limit to 75 calories/
315 kilojoules per day)**
Chewing gum, sugar-free
Cocoa powder, unsweetened
Jelly, sugar-free
Lollipops, sugar-free
Sugar substitute
Sweets, hard, sugar-free

Foods to Avoid

BEEF
Fatty cuts, such as:
Brisket
Rib roasts

LAMB
Fatty cuts such as shoulder
Liver

PORK

Honey-baked ham

Sausages

POULTRY

Chicken, wings and legs

Duck

Goose

Poultry products, processed

CHEESE

Avoid full-fat cheeses,
including:

Brie

Edam

VEGETABLES

Beetroot

Carrots

Jerusalem artichokes

Potatoes, sweet

Potatoes, white

Sweetcorn

Yams

FRUIT

Avoid all fruits and fruit juices
in Phase 1

STARCHES

Avoid all starchy food in
Phase 1, including:

Bread (all types)

Cereal

Matzo

Oats

Pasta (all types)

Pastry and baked goods (all
types

Rice (all types)

DAIRY

Ice cream

Milk, whole (full-fat) or semi-
skimmed (low-fat)

Sweetened soya milk

Yogurt, regular or frozen

MISCELLANEOUS

Avoid alcohol of any kind in
Phase 1, including beer and
wine

Phase 2

As with Phase 1, Phase 2 also has recommendations for which foods to eat. The first list tells you which foods to reintroduce into your diet. The second list includes foods that you'd best eat only rarely – any more than that could affect your blood glucose levels and derail your weight-loss efforts as well.

Foods You Can Reintroduce to Your Diet

VEGETABLES AND PULSES
Carrots
Peas, green
Potato, small, sweet

STARCHES (limit)
Bagels, small, wholemeal
Barley
Bread
   multigrain
   oat and bran
   rye
   wholemeal
Cereal
   high-fibre, low-sugar cereals
   porridge (not quick-cooking)

Pasta, wholewheat
Pitta bread
   stoneground
   wholemeal
Popcorn (air-popped)
Rice
   brown
   wild

FRUIT
Apples
Apricots, dried or fresh
Blueberries
Cherries
Grapefruit
Grapes
Kiwi fruit

Mangoes

Melons, green-, orange- and yellow-fleshed

Oranges

Peaches

Pears

Plums

Strawberries

MISCELLANEOUS

Chocolate, plain, dark (look for high cocoa solids and eat sparingly)

Dessert, fat-free, sugar-free

Wine, red or white

Foods to Avoid or Eat Rarely

VEGETABLES

Beetroot

Potatoes, white

Sweetcorn

STARCHES

Bagel, white flour

Biscuits

Bread and rolls, brown or white

Cornflakes

Matzo

Pasta, white

Rice cakes

Rice, white

FRUIT

Bananas

Canned fruit, juice-packed

Fruit juice

Pineapple

Raisins

Watermelon

MISCELLANEOUS

Honey

Ice cream

Jam

How about refined, bad carbs? Not surprisingly, their processed sugars enter the bloodstream quickly. This makes insulin rise quickly, followed by a rapid fall in blood sugar.

On the South Beach Diet, you'll tend to eat foods that fall lower on the GI, prepared or eaten in ways that allow your body to digest and absorb them more slowly. After Phase 1, the strictest phase of the Diet, you'll reintroduce good carbohydrates with a higher GI.

While the GI is an astounding breakthrough in our understanding of how carbohydrates affect our metabolism, there are a few important things you need to know to use the system successfully. First, the GI doesn't account for portion size. The solution: the concept of the glycaemic load (GL), which takes into account a food's GI (the quality of carbohydrate) as well as the amount (the quantity of carbohydrate) per serving. It also represents the load, or stress, placed on the pancreas from the amount of carbohydrates consumed from a particular food or meal.

For this Guide, our evaluation of each food choice is based on the glycaemic index, glycaemic load, and on other factors as well. Our recommendations are meant to be guidelines, not absolute do's and don'ts. As we learn more, there will certainly be changes in future editions.

A good diet is always a work in progress, because scientists are always conducting new research. In reading this guide, you will notice that our recommendations on a few key foods have changed since the original South Beach Diet book was published. Specifically, we now allow you to eat as many tomatoes as you want, even in Phase 1. Though technically a fruit, tomatoes have a low GI and contain a lot of nutrients. Carrots, too, are now allowed in Phase 2, because of new research on their glycaemic index value. Finally, and for many of you most importantly, our recommendation on dairy products has changed. Although milk contains some sugars in the form of lactose, recent studies have shown that lactose may help control body fat. Whole milk is not allowed as it is high in saturated fat, but you can enjoy skimmed milk and fat-free natural yogurt in Phase 1. To keep abreast of all changes and new recommendations for the diet, visit *www.southbeachdiet.com/updates* regularly.

HOW TO USE
THE FOOD GUIDE

The South Beach Diet doesn't require you to count calories or fat or carbohydrate grams. But bad carbs and bad fats have a way of sneaking up on you, especially when you're dining out or eating on the run. This Guide gives you the knowledge you need to make healthy food choices. Use it faithfully and you'll be virtually guaranteed to stick to South Beach principles – anytime, anywhere.

The more than 1,300 foods in this Guide are listed in alphabetical order by category. Each entry lists the total amount of carbohydrates, sugar and fat for one portion. In the last column is our recommendation for how to incorporate this food into your diet. This recommendation is based on many factors, including the glycaemic index, the glycaemic load, the fibre and nutrient content of the food, and more.

Within specific categories, the recommendation assigned to each food is usually either 'Good', 'Limited', 'Very Limited', or 'Avoid'. In a few instances, we use 'Allowed', for foods where implying quantities might be misleading. Sugar substitutes are one example of that. But it's possible that the foods available in your supermarket are different from those we've analysed, even if it's the same *type* of food. So remember to read the labels! Watch out for tinned foods thickened with cornflour or other starches, powdered mixes that contain trans fats (see page 8), and sugar additives such as glucose syrup.

These recommendations are guidelines, not hard and fast rules, because so much depends on you as an individual. How often you might eat something depends on which Phase of the diet you are on, how much weight you're trying to lose, your body's own metabolism, and so on. Certain categories of foods, such as whole fruits, are identified as 'good' because they are in fact good, healthy foods, but if you're in Phase 1 of the diet you still need to avoid them entirely (see pages 22–23). When you do reintroduce more good carbs in Phase 2 (see pages 24–25) and beyond, do so with discretion and pay attention to how your body responds. The South Beach Diet is not just a way of eating; it's a way of thinking about food. Once you understand its principles, you'll always be able to make the right food choices.

Tr = Trace

1 tsp = 5 ml

1 tbsp = 15 ml

BEANS AND PULSES

Beans and pulses are excellent sources of soluble fibre, which delays stomach emptying time, slows glucose absorption, and can lower blood cholesterol and assist weight loss. Beans are also an excellent source of protein for vegetarians. For bean sprouts, broad beans and green beans, turn to the Vegetables and Herbs section on page 125.

Soya protein, found in soya beans and soya products, lowers LDL (bad) cholesterol. We recommend liberal consumption of these healthy foods.

Avoid canned beans that contain sugar and/or salt.

Food	Portion	Total Carbs (g)	Total Sugar (g)	Total Fat (g)	Recmmd.
Aduki beans, boiled	60 g (2 oz)	14	0.5	0	Good
Baked beans					
in tomato sauce	90 g (3 oz)	14	5	0.5	Good
w/meatballs, canned	90 g (3 oz)	11	3	3.5	Very Limited
w/pork sausages, canned	90 g (3 oz)	10	4	2	Very Limited
w/vegetarian sausages, canned	90 g (3 oz)	11	4	3	Very Limited
Black beans, boiled	60 g (2 oz)	12	1	0.5	Good
Black-eyed beans, canned, drained	60 g (2 oz)	11	1	0.5	Good
Borlotti beans, canned, drained	60 g (2 oz)	11	1	0.5	Good
Butter beans, canned, drained	60 g (2 oz)	8	1	0.5	Good
Cannellini beans, canned, drained	60 g (2 oz)	8	2	0.5	Good

BEANS AND PULSES (CONT.)

Food	Portion	Total Carbs (g)	Total Sugar (g)	Total Fat (g)	Recmmd.
Chickpeas, canned, drained	60 g (2 oz)	10	0.5	2	Good
Chilli beans, canned	90 g (3 oz)	15	3	0.5	Good
Chilli, vegetarian, with soya mince	90 g (3 oz)	12	4	2.5	Good
Chilli con carne, canned	90 g (3 oz)	4	2.5	7	Avoid
Edamame (green soya beans), fresh or frozen	60 g (2 oz)	7	1	4	Good
Flageolet beans, canned, drained	60 g (2 oz)	10	1	0.5	Good
Haricot beans, boiled	60 g (2 oz)	10	1	0.5	Good
Kidney beans, red, canned or boiled	60 g (2 oz)	11	2	0.5	Good
Lentils, brown, green or red, boiled	60 g (2 oz)	10	0.5	0.5	Good
Mung beans, cooked	60 g (2 oz)	9	0.5	0.5	Good
Pinto beans, boiled	60 g (2 oz)	9	0.5	0.5	Good

Food	Portion	Total Carbs (g)	Total Sugar (g)	Total Fat (g)	Recmmd.
Refried beans					
fat-free, canned	90 g (3 oz)	11	1	Tr	Good
regular, canned	90 g (3 oz)	12	1	1	Good
Soya beans, canned	60 g (2 oz)	3	1	4	Good

PEAS

Food	Portion	Total Carbs (g)	Total Sugar (g)	Total Fat (g)	Recmmd.
Green peas, fresh or frozen	60 g (2 oz)	7	1.5	1	Limited
Mangetouts (snow peas), raw	60 g (2 oz)	2.5	2	0	Good
Mushy peas, canned	90 g (3 oz)	12	1.5	0.5	Limited
Peas, canned	60 g (2 oz)	8	2	0.5	Limited
Split peas, boiled	60 g (2 oz)	10	Tr	0.5	Good
Sugar snap peas, fresh or frozen	60 g (2 oz)	2.5	2	0.5	Good

BREAD AND BREAD PRODUCTS

Like other grain products, breads can be enjoyed often if you choose the right ones. Wholegrain and multigrain breads are the best choice. Wholegrain products should be labelled '100 per cent whole wheat', 'whole oats' or 'whole rye'. Other good choices are sourdough bread and wholegrain pumpernickel.

By law, products made with white and brown flour are fortified with certain nutrients – because processing has removed essential vitamins and minerals. Any attempts to return nutrients artificially are unlikely to be sufficient. Breads that are labelled 'wholemeal' retain all their nutrients but the glycaemic index is generally just as high as that of white bread. Look for at least 3 grams of fibre per serving. Avoid commercial breads that include hydrogenated oils.

Remember, according to the guidelines for Phase 2, you should moderate your consumption of all breads and starches once they are reintroduced to your diet.

Food	Portion	Total Carbs (g)	Total Sugar (g)	Total Fat (g)	Recmmd.
Bagels					
Blueberry	85 g (3 oz)	44	8	1.5	Avoid
Cinnamon and raisin	85 g (3 oz)	44	6	2	Avoid
Plain	85 g (3 oz)	49	5.5	1.5	Avoid
Sesame	85 g (3 oz)	45	2	2	Avoid
Onion and poppyseed	85 g (3 oz)	45	2	2	Avoid
Multigrain	115 g (4 oz)	45	2	1	Avoid
Bread					
Baguette, white	5 cm (2 in) slice	22	1	1	Avoid
Ciabatta	75 g (2½ oz)	39	2.5	3	Avoid

Food	Portion	Total Carbs (g)	Total Sugar (g)	Total Fat (g)	Recmmd.
Cinnamon raisin	1 slice 40 g (1¼ oz)	20	11	5	Avoid
Focaccia	50 g (1¾ oz)	22	2	6	Avoid
Granary	1 slice 30 g (1 oz)	14	1	1	Very Limited
Gluten-free, wheat-free	1 slice 30 g (1 oz)	14	1	1	Very Limited
Honey oat	1 slice 30 g (1 oz)	13	1	1	Very Limited
Malt loaf, fruited	1 slice 30 g (1 oz)	20	7	1	Very Limited
Multigrain	1 slice 30 g (1 oz)	14	1	1	Limited
Naan, plain	½ naan 75 g (2½ oz)	35	2	6	Very Limited
Naan, filled	½ naan 75 g (2½ oz)	33	1	10	Avoid
Oatmeal	1 slice 45 g (1½ oz)	22	4	2	Limited
Pitta, wholemeal	15 cm (6 in) pitta	38	1	2	Limited
Pitta, white	15 cm (6 in) pitta	41	2	1	Limited
Potato and rosemary	1 slice, 30 g (1 oz)	14	1	1	Avoid
Pumpernickel, wholegrain	1 slice 50 g (1¾ oz)	24	0.5	1.5	Limited
Rye, light	1 slice, 30 g (1 oz)	14	0.5	0.5	Limited

BREAD AND BREAD PRODUCTS (CONT.)

Food	Portion	Total Carbs (g)	Total Sugar (g)	Total Fat (g)	Recmmd.
Soda bread	1 'farl', 115 g (4 oz)	50	4	4	Avoid
Sourdough, rye	1 slice, 60 g (2 oz)	31	0.5	2	Limited
Sourdough, wheat	1 slice, 60 g (2 oz)	31	0.5	2	Limited
Soya and linseed	1 slice 30 g (1 oz)	10	0.5	2	Limited
Stoneground wholewheat	1 slice 30 g (1 oz)	13	1	1	Limited
Sunflower and barley	1 slice	12	0.5	2	Limited
Tapioca bread	1 slice 30 g	14	1	1	Limited
White	1 slice 30 g (1 oz)	14	1	0.5	Avoid
Wholemeal	1 slice 30 g	13	1	1	Limited
Muffins					
White	1 muffin 65 g	29	2	1	Very Limited
Wholemeal	1 muffin 65 g	28	2	1	Limited

BREAD PRODUCTS

Food	Portion	Total Carbs (g)	Total Sugar (g)	Total Fat (g)	Recmmd.
Breadcrumbs					
Dry, plain	30 g (1 oz)	17	1	1	Avoid
Gluten-free, wheat-free	30 g (1 oz)	14	1	0.5	Avoid

Food	Portion	Total Carbs (g)	Total Sugar (g)	Total Fat (g)	Recmmd.
Fresh, white	30 g (1 oz)	14	1	0.5	Avoid
Breadsticks, plain	1 breadstick	5	0.5	0.5	Avoid
Bread stuffing, prepared	60 g (2 oz)	17	2.5	9	Avoid
Croutons, plain, dry	15 g (½ oz)	11	1	1	Avoid
Crumpet	1 crumpet	18	1	0.5	Avoid
Rolls					
Brioche	1 brioche 50 g (1¾ oz)	26	1	1	Avoid
Cheese-topped	1 roll 60 g (2 oz)	30	1.5	2	Avoid
Frankfurter/hot dog roll	1 roll 90 g (3 oz)	46	2.5	2.5	Very Limited
Hamburger bun	1 bun 60 g (2 oz)	29	1	3	Very Limited
Potato scone	40 g (1¼ oz)	14	4	0.5	Avoid
Soft white roll	50 g (1¾ oz)	26	1	1	Avoid
Floury bap	50 g (1¾ oz)	26	1	1	Avoid
Granary roll	75 g (2½ oz)	32	2	3	Limited
Taco shell, baked	1 taco 15 g	9	1	4	Avoid
Tortilla (soft) corn	1 tortilla 40 g	18	1	4	Very Limited
Tortilla (soft) wheat flour	1 tortilla 30 g	16	1	2	Limited

BREAKFAST FOODS

Man was designed to consume much more fibre than we get in modern diets. Fibre slows our digestion and thereby helps prevent swings in our sugar and insulin levels. Both hot and cold breakfast cereals can be excellent sources of fibre; choose ones with at least 6 g of fibre per 100 g. Porridge and hot oat cereals can be excellent, but only those that are slow cooked; instant hot cereals have high glycaemic indices. And don't be fooled by cereals labelled 'natural'. Many types, including muesli, have plenty of sugar and minimal fibre. Even worse, they may contain hydrogenated oils (trans fats) – the worst type of fats.

Sweet pastries, doughnuts and shop-bought muffins are the worst breakfast choice. They have high levels of trans fats and highly processed flour, are usually loaded with sugars, and have a very high glycaemic index.

CEREAL BARS

Food	Portion	Total Carbs (g)	Total Sugar (g)	Total Fat (g)	Recmmd.
Chewy bar	27 g	17	9	4	Avoid
Crunchy bar	33 g	20	9	7	Avoid
Frusli	33 g	22	13	3	Avoid
Nutri-Grain	37 g	26	11	3	Avoid
Tracker	27 g	16	9	7	Avoid
Uncle Tobys	32 g	20	7	3	Avoid

CEREALS, COLD, DRY

Food	Portion	Total Carbs (g)	Total Sugar (g)	Total Fat (g)	Recmmd.
All-Bran	40 g (1¼ oz)	19	8	1.5	Good
High Fibre Bran	30 g (1 oz)	18	1	1	Good
Bran Flakes	30 g (1 oz)	21	7	1	Limited
Cheerios	40 g (1¼ oz)	32	9	1.5	Limited
Corn Flakes	30 g (1 oz)	27	2.5	0.5	Avoid
Corn Pops	40 g (1¼ oz)	35	14	1	Avoid

Food	Portion	Total Carbs (g)	Total Sugar (g)	Total Fat (g)	Recmmd.
Force	40 g (1¼ oz)	28	3	1	Limited
Frosties	30 g (1 oz)	28	13	Tr	Avoid
Fruit and Fibre	30 g (1 oz)	22	7	1.5	Very Limited
Golden Grahams	40 g (1¼ oz)	32	13	1	Avoid
Grape Nuts	30 g (1 oz)	22	4	0.5	Avoid
Honey Loops	30 g (1 oz)	23	10	1	Avoid
Just Right	45 g (1½ oz)	32	14	Tr	Avoid
Kashi	30 g (1 oz)	22	0	1	Good
Muesli					
Swiss style (e.g. Alpen)	40 g (1¼ oz)	29	11	2	Avoid
Swiss, unsweetened	40 g (1¼ oz)	27	6	3	Limited
w/honey and almonds	50 g (1¾ oz)	31	12	9	Avoid
w/coconut and tropical fruit	50 g (1¾ oz)	33	11	7	Avoid
Oat crunch	40 g (1¼ oz)	26	11	5	Avoid
Puffed wheat	30 g (1 oz)	20	Tr	Tr	Avoid
Rice Krispies (Rice Bubbles)	30 g (1 oz)	28	3	Tr	Avoid
Ricicles	30 g (1 oz)	28	13	Tr	Avoid
Shredded Wheat	2 biscuits	32	Tr	1	Limited
Shreddies	50 g (1¾ oz)	39	8	1	Avoid
Special K	30 g (1 oz)	25	5	Tr	Limited
Start multigrain	30 g (1 oz)	25	10	1	Limited

BREAKFAST FOODS (CONT.)

Food	Portion	Total Carbs (g)	Total Sugar (g)	Total Fat (g)	Recmmd.
Sugar Puffs	30 g (1 oz)	28	15	Tr	Avoid
Sultana Bran	45 g (1½ oz)	28	10	Tr	Very Limited
Weetabix (Weet-Bix)	2 biscuits	32	2	1	Limited

CEREALS, HOT, PREPARED WITH WATER

Food	Portion	Total Carbs (g)	Total Sugar (g)	Total Fat (g)	Recmmd.
Millet	30 g (1 oz)	7	0	Tr	Avoid
Porridge and oat cereals					
Oat bran	30 g (1 oz)	15	0.5	2	Good
Oat cereal, instant	30 g (1 oz)	20	0.5	2.5	Avoid
Oat cereal, instant, flavoured	40 g (1¼ oz)	21	1	2.5	Avoid
Porridge oats, traditional	50 g (1¾ oz)	30	Tr	4	Good
Porridge oats, quick-cooking	30 g (1 oz)	20	Tr	3	Limited

CEREAL TOPPINGS

Food	Portion	Total Carbs (g)	Total Sugar (g)	Total Fat (g)	Recmmd.
Almonds	6 nuts	1	0.5	6	Good
Honey	1 tbsp	19	19	0	Very Limited
Oat bran, unprocessed	2 tbsp	10	Tr	1	Good

Food	Portion	Total Carbs (g)	Total Sugar (g)	Total Fat (g)	Recmmd.
Psyllium	1 tbsp	2	0.5	0.5	Good
Raisins	2 tbsp	42	42	Tr	Very Limited
Sugar	1 tsp	5	5	0	Very Limited
Wheat bran	2 tbsp	5	1	1	Good
Wheat germ	1 tbsp	4	1	2	Good

FAST FOOD BREAKFAST MUFFINS

Food	Portion	Total Carbs (g)	Total Sugar (g)	Total Fat (g)	Recmmd.
Bacon and egg	1 muffin (145 g)	26	1	18	Avoid
Egg	1 muffin (125 g)	26	1	13	Avoid
Sausage and egg	1 muffin (175 g)	26	1	25	Avoid

PANCAKES AND PASTRIES

Food	Portion	Total Carbs (g)	Total Sugar (g)	Total Fat (g)	Recmmd.
Croissants					
Plain	1 medium, 50 g (1¾ oz)	22	3	10	Avoid
Cheese	1 medium	22	3	11	Avoid
Ham and cheese	100 g (3½ oz)	8	3	11	Avoid
Danish pastries					
Apple and sultana	1 pastry 75 g	34	19	13	Avoid
Pecan	1 pastry 65 g	31	17	17	Avoid

BREAKFAST FOODS (CONT.)

Food	Portion	Total Carbs (g)	Total Sugar (g)	Total Fat (g)	Recmmd.
Plain	1 pastry 110 g	56	31	15	Avoid
95% fat-free apple and cinnamon Danish twist	60 g (2 oz)	30	16	3	Avoid
Doughnuts					
Apple-filled	110 g (4 oz)	43	23	20	Avoid
Custard-filled	75 g (2½ oz)	22	11	15	Avoid
Jam-filled	75 g (2½ oz)	37	14	11	Avoid
Ring	75 g (2½ oz)	35	11	17	Avoid
Ring w/icing	75 g (2½ oz)	38	18	16	Avoid
Muffins					
Blueberry	75 g (2½ oz)	40	9	7	Avoid
Bran	60 g (2 oz)	29	5	5	Avoid
Chocolate chip	75 g (2½ oz)	40	21	14	Avoid
Cinnamon and raisin (English-type	1 muffin 65 g (2 oz)	32	13	2	Avoid
Lemon and poppyseed	1 muffin 60 g (2 oz)	28	11	2	Avoid
Low-fat	60 g (2 oz)	31	6	2	Avoid
White (English-type)	1 muffin 65 g (2 oz)	29	2	1	Very Limited
Wholemeal (English-type)	1 muffin 65 g (2 oz)	28	2	1	Limited
Pain au chocolat	60 g (2 oz)	27	6	12	Avoid

Food	Portion	Total Carbs (g)	Total Sugar (g)	Total Fat (g)	Recmmd.
Pancakes					
Scotch	30 g (1 oz)	13	6	3	Avoid
Sultana and syrup	40 g (1¼ oz)	14	8	2	Avoid
Apple and sultana	75 g (2½ oz)	40	23	6	Avoid
Pop tarts					
Chocolate	1	35	17	6	Avoid
Brown sugar and cinnamon	1	36	17	6	Avoid
Strawberry	1	36	16	6	Avoid
Potato scones	1 small 40 g (1¼ oz)	14	4	0.5	Avoid

CAKES AND BISCUITS

Many food manufacturers add hydrogenated (or partially hydrogenated) fats – trans fats – to replace the previously used saturated fats as a way of extending products' shelf lives. Trans fats are common in commercial cakes, biscuits and baking mixes. Trans fats are worse than saturated fats and should be avoided as much as possible.

CAKES

Food	Portion	Total Carbs (g)	Total Sugar (g)	Total Fat (g)	Recmmd.
Banana bread	60 g (2 oz)	32	22	8	Avoid
Madeira cake	60 g (2 oz)	35	22	9	Avoid
Cheesecake, plain	75 g (2½ oz)	26	19	10	Avoid
Chocolate cake, w/chocolate icing	75 g (2½ oz)	42	33	11	Avoid
Chocolate eclair	60 g (2 oz)	16	4	18	Avoid

CAKES (CONT.)

Food	Portion	Total Carbs (g)	Total Sugar (g)	Total Fat (g)	Recmmd.
Coffee cake, w/nuts	1 slice, 60 g (2 oz)	26	15	7	Avoid
Ginger cake	1 slice, 40 g (1¼ oz)	23	15	6	Avoid
Malt loaf	1 slice, 30 g (1 oz)	20	7	1	Very Limited
Plain fruit cake	1 slice, 90 g (3 oz)	52	39	13	Avoid
Scone, plain	1 40 g (1¼ oz)	21	2	6	Avoid
Scone, fruit	1 40 g (1¼ oz)	22	8	4	Avoid
Sponge cake, plain	1 slice, 60 g (2 oz)	31	18	16	Avoid
Strudel, apple	1 slice, 100 g (3½ oz)	41	26	11	Avoid
Swiss roll, w/jam	1 slice, 20 g (¾ oz)	13	10	1	Avoid
Teacake	1, 60 g (2 oz)	35	10	5	Avoid
Victoria sandwich	1 slice 60 g (2 oz)	26	15	6	Avoid

BISCUITS

Food	Portion	Total Carbs (g)	Total Sugar (g)	Total Fat (g)	Recmmd.
Chocolate sandwich biscuit (e.g. Bourbon)	1 biscuit	9	5	3	Avoid
Custard cream	1 biscuit	11	5	3	Avoid
Digestive (wheatmeal)	1 biscuit	10	2	3	Avoid
Fig roll	1 roll	13	7	1	Avoid
Garibaldi	1 biscuit	7	3	1	Avoid
Gingernut biscuits	2 small biscuits	19	9	3	Avoid
Jaffa cake	1	9	6	1	Avoid
Milk chocolate-coated finger	2 fingers	8	5	3	Avoid
Oat-based biscuit (e.g. Hob Nobs)	1 biscuit	9	4	4	Avoid
Oat flapjack	1, 40 g (1¼ oz)	25	14	11	Avoid
Sweet biscuit (e.g. Nice)	1 biscuit	6	2	1	Avoid
Semi-sweet biscuit (e.g. Marie, Rich Tea)	1 biscuit	7	2	1	Avoid
Shortbread	1 finger	8	2	4	Avoid

CHEESE AND CHEESE PRODUCTS

Whole milk cheeses are a source of saturated fat, so choose low-fat or fat-free cheese for most of your eating and snacking. Mozzarella cheese sticks make convenient and healthy snacks. Occasionally, however, it's OK to enjoy a small amount of a very flavourful cheese such as blue cheese, feta, goat's cheese or Parmesan, because a little goes a long way to enhance the flavour of a dish without contributing too much saturated fat.

CHEESE

Food	Portion	Total Carbs (g)	Total Sugar (g)	Total Fat (g)	Recmmd.
Blue cheese	30 g (1 oz)	0	0	11	Limited
Brie	30 g (1 oz)	0	0	9	Avoid
Half-fat	30 g (1 oz)	0	0	4.5	Limited
Camembert	30 g (1 oz)	0	0	7	Avoid
Cheddar					
3% fat	30 g (1 oz)	0	0	1	Good
Half-fat	30 g (1 oz)	0	0	5	Limited
Regular	30 g (1 oz)	0	0	10	Avoid
Cheshire	30 g (1 oz)	0	0	10	Avoid
Cottage cheese					
Virtually fat-free	115 g (4 oz)	8	8	0.5	Good
Low-fat (1.5% fat)	115 g (4 oz)	8	8	1.5	Limited
Creamed, less than 3% fat	115 g (4 oz)	6	6	3.5	Very Limited
Regular (4% fat)	115 g (4 oz)	5	5	4.5	Avoid
Cream cheese					
Light	30 g (1 oz)	1	1	2	Good
Regular	30 g (1 oz)	0	0	10	Avoid

Food	Portion	Total Carbs (g)	Total Sugar (g)	Total Fat (g)	Recmmd.
Double Gloucester	30 g (1 oz)	0	0	10	Avoid
Edam	30 g (1 oz)	0	0	8	Avoid
Reduced-fat	30 g (1 oz)	0	0	4	Limited
Emmental	30 g (1 oz)	0	0	9	Avoid
Reduced-fat	30 g (1 oz)	1	1	2	Good
Feta	30 g (1 oz)	0.5	0.5	6	Limited
Fromage frais					
Virtually fat-free	100 g (3½ oz)	5	4	Tr	Good
Regular	100 g (3½ oz)	4	4	8	Limited
w/fruit, sweetened	100 g (3½ oz)	14	13	6	Avoid
Goat's cheese					
Hard	30 g (1 oz)	0	0	9	Limited
Soft	30 g (1 oz)	0	0	8	Limited
Gorgonzola	30 g (1 oz)	0	0	9	Avoid
Gouda	30 g (1 oz)	Tr	Tr	9	Avoid
Gruyère	30 g (1 oz)	Tr	Tr	10	Avoid
Halloumi	30 g (1 oz)	1	1	7	Avoid
Jarlsberg	30 g (1 oz)	0	0	8	Avoid
Lancashire	30 g (1 oz)	0	0	9	Avoid
Mascarpone	30 g (1 oz)	1.5	1.5	12	Avoid
Mozzarella					
Buffalo milk	30 g (1 oz)	0	0	8	Good
Light	30 g (1 oz)	0.5	0.5	3	Good
Whole milk	30 g (1 oz)	0.5	0.5	6	Limited

CHEESE AND CHEESE PRODUCTS (CONT.)

Food	Portion	Total Carbs (g)	Total Sugar (g)	Total Fat (g)	Recmmd.
Parmesan	30 g (1 oz)	Tr	Tr	9	Limited
Parmesan, grated	1 tbsp	Tr	Tr	5	Good
Pecorino (hard, sheep's milk)	30 g (1 oz)	0	0	9	Avoid
Port Salut	30 g (1 oz)	Tr	Tr	8	Avoid
Quark	100 g (3½ oz)	4	4	Tr	Limited
Ricotta	30 g (1 oz)	1	1	3	Good
Roquefort	30 g (1 oz)	0	0	10	Limited
Stilton	30 g (1 oz)	Tr	Tr	10	Limited

CHEESE PRODUCTS

Food	Portion	Total Carbs (g)	Total Sugar (g)	Total Fat (g)	Recmmd.
Cheese slices					
Skimmed milk (97% fat-free)	1 slice	1	1	0.5	Good
Light	1 slice	1	1	3	Limited
Regular	1 slice	1	1	5	Limited
Cheese spread					
w/chilli	30 g (1 oz)	1	1	6	Avoid
Light	30 g (1 oz)	1	1	2	Avoid
Regular	30 g (1 oz)	1	1	6	Avoid
Cheese triangles					
Light	1	Tr	Tr	2	Limited
Regular	1	Tr	Tr	4	Limited

Food	Portion	Total Carbs (g)	Total Sugar (g)	Total Fat (g)	Recmmd.
Garlic and herb soft cheese					
Benecol	30 g (1 oz)	1	1	4	Good
Light	30 g (1 oz)	1	1	2	Good
Regular	30 g (1 oz)	1	1	5	Limited
Soya cheese	30 g (1 oz)	1	0	9	Good
String cheese	30 g (1 oz)	Tr	Tr	7	Limited

CONFECTIONERY

Most sweets are made from sugar and unhealthy fats, and as such should be avoided. However, if you are going to indulge, a small quantity of plain dark chocolate with a high percentage of cocoa solids is the best choice: this has a lower sugar content than other types of chocolate.

There are now many varieties of low-carb, sugar-free and diabetic sweets on the market. Many use sugar alcohols such as sorbitol or xylitol as sweeteners. These taste sweet, but instead of being absorbed into the bloodstream, they pass through the intestines. Consuming sweets made with these sweeteners can cause stomach upset and diarrhoea.

Food	Portion	Total Carbs (g)	Total Sugar (g)	Total Fat (g)	Recmmd.
Boiled sweets and clear mints	1 sweet (5 g)	4	4	0	Avoid
Boiled sweets, sugar-free	1 sweet (5 g)	4	0	0	Limited
Chewing gum, sugar-free	1 stick	4	0	0	Limited
Chocolate					
Fruit and nut	30 g (1 oz)	16	15	9	Avoid
Milk	30 g (1 oz)	17	17	9	Avoid

CONFECTIONERY (CONT.)

Food	Portion	Total Carbs (g)	Total Sugar (g)	Total Fat (g)	Recmmd.
Plain	30 g (1 oz)	19	18	8	Avoid
Plain, 70% cocoa solids	30 g (1 oz)	8	7	14	Very Limited
Chocolate peanuts	30 g (1 oz)	13	7	10	Very Limited
Chocolate raisins	30 g (1 oz)	19	13	6	Avoid
Fruit leather	15 g (½ oz)	12	9	0	Limited
Fudge	30 g (1 oz)	24	24	4	Avoid
Gums and jelly sweets					
Fruit gums	30 g (1 oz)	24	18	0	Avoid
Jelly babies	30 g (1 oz)	23	21	0	Avoid
Wine gums	30 g (1 oz)	23	19	0	Avoid
Liquorice All Sorts	60 g (2 oz)	46	37	2	Avoid
Marshmallows, regular-size	2 pieces	12	10	0	Avoid
Mars bar	42 g	33	28	8	Avoid
Polo mints, sugar-free	30 g (1 oz)	10	0	0	Avoid
Rolos	1 Rolo	6	5	2	Avoid
Toffee apple	1	24	21	3	Avoid
Toffee popcorn	30 g (1 oz)	23	19	5	Avoid
Yogurt-coated fruit	30 g (1 oz)	22	20	5	Avoid
Yogurt-coated nuts	30 g (1 oz)	12	11	11	Avoid

CRACKERS, CRISPBREADS, SNACKS AND DIPS

Most crackers and packaged snack foods contain trans fats and should be avoided.

CRACKERS

Food	Portion	Total Carbs (g)	Total Sugar (g)	Total Fat (g)	Recmmd.
Bath Oliver	1	8	Tr	2	Avoid
Cheese-flavoured crackers	1	4	1	2	Avoid
Cornish wafer	1	2	0.5	1	Avoid
Cream cracker	1	5	Tr	1	Avoid
Crispbread, rye	1	4	Tr	Tr	Avoid
Crispbread, rye, high fibre	1	4	Tr	Tr	Limited
Digestive biscuit, plain (wheatmeal)	1	10	2	3	Avoid
Matzo crackers	2	6	0	Tr	Avoid
Melba toast	1	4	Tr	Tr	Avoid
Rice cake					
Flavoured	1	6	Tr	Tr	Avoid
Plain	1	6	Tr	Tr	Very Limited
Ritz crackers	2	4	Tr	2	Avoid
Sandwich cracker, w/cheese filling	1	5	1	3	Avoid
High bake water biscuit	1	12	Tr	1	Avoid
Scottish oatcake	1	7	0.5	2	Limited

CRACKERS, CRISPBREADS, SNACKS AND DIPS (CONT.)

Food	Portion	Total Carbs (g)	Total Sugar (g)	Total Fat (g)	Recmmd.
Water crackers	4	8	0.5	1.5	Avoid
Wheaten cracker	1	4	Tr	2	Avoid

DIPS

Food	Portion	Total Carbs (g)	Total Sugar (g)	Total Fat (g)	Recmmd.
Aubergine (eggplant)	2 tbsp	2	1	10	Good
Blue cheese	2 tbsp	2	1	15	Avoid
Cheese and chive	2 tbsp	1.5	0.5	13	Avoid
Garlic and herb	2 tbsp	1.5	0.5	12	Avoid
Onion and garlic	2 tbsp	1.5	1	12	Avoid
Guacamole (avocado dip)	2 tbsp	1	0.5	6	Good
Hummus	2 tbsp	4	Tr	6	Good
Reduced-fat	2 tbsp	4	Tr	4	Good
Chunky salsa	2 tbsp	4	3	1	Good
Sour cream and chive	2 tbsp	1	0.5	11	Avoid
Taramasalata	2 tbsp	2	0.5	14	Avoid
Tzatziki (cucumber and yogurt)	2 tbsp	0.5	0.5	1.5	Limited

SNACKS

Food	Portion	Total Carbs (g)	Total Sugar (g)	Total Fat (g)	Recmmd.
Banana chips	30 g (1 oz)	17	10	10	Avoid
Bombay mix	50 g (1¾ oz)	17	1	16	Avoid
Cheese puffs or cheese curls	1 small pack (20 g)	11	2	6	Avoid
Corn snacks	1 small pack (20 g)	11	1	7	Avoid
Dried fruit bar	1 (35 g)	24	15	Tr	Avoid
Hula Hoops	1 small pack (30 g)	17	Tr	8	Avoid
Olives					
Black, pitted	30 g (1 oz)	2	Tr	5	Good
Black, stuffed, in brine	30 g (1 oz)	1	Tr	5	Good
Green, pitted	30 g (1 oz)	1.5	Tr	5	Good
Green, stuffed, in brine	30 g (1 oz)	1	Tr	5	Good
Green, stuffed, in oil	30 g (1 oz)	1	Tr	8	Good
Popcorn					
Air-popped, plain	30 g (1 oz)	21	2	5	Limited
Air-popped, w/1 tsp butter	30 g (1 oz)	19	2	7	Avoid
Air-popped, w/1 tsp oil	30 g (1 oz)	19	2	7	Limited
Microwave popcorn, plain	30 g (1 oz)	21	2	5	Avoid

CRACKERS, CRISPBREADS, SNACKS AND DIPS (CONT.)

Food	Portion	Total Carbs (g)	Total Sugar (g)	Total Fat (g)	Recmmd.
Poppadum snacks	30 g (1 oz)	11	0.5	10	Avoid
Potato crisps (chips)					
Plain	30 g (1 oz)	16	Tr	10	Avoid
Flavoured	30 g (1 oz)	16	Tr	10	Avoid
Reduced- or low fat	30 g (1 oz)	18	0.5	6	Avoid
Potato sticks	30 g (1 oz)	19	Tr	5	Avoid
Prawn crackers	15 g (½ oz)	9	Tr	5	Avoid
Pretzels					
Fat-free	50 g (1¾ oz)	41	1	0.5	Avoid
Regular	50 g (1¾ oz)	40	1	2.5	Avoid
Pringles					
Original	50 g (1¾ oz)	24	0.5	19	Avoid
Flavoured	50 g (1¾ oz)	24	1	18	Avoid
Tortilla chips	40 g (1¼ oz)	24	0.5	9	Avoid
Trail mix, w/raisins and nuts	30 g (1 oz)	11	11	8	Avoid

DESERTS

Desserts are fairly limited on Phase 1 of the South Beach Diet, although you can feel free to enjoy sugar-free jelly, unsweetened and fat-free yogurt or fromage frais, and ricotta – to which you may add sugar substitute, unsweetened cocoa powder, vanilla extract, or a few almonds.

Fruits, particularly berries, are ideal Phase 2 desserts. Strawberries dipped in dark chocolate are a personal favourite! Remember, the darker the chocolate, the lower the sugar content.

JELLY

Food	Portion	Total Carbs (g)	Total Sugar (g)	Total Fat (g)	Recmmd.
Sugar-free, prepared from crystals	1 sachet (25 g)	Tr	Tr	0	Good
w/fruit, prepared, ready-to eat	1 pot, 170 g (6 oz)	27	27	0	Avoid
w/sugar, prepared from cubes	¼ jelly, 145 g (5 oz)	22	22	0	Avoid

PASTRY, PIES AND TARTS

Food	Portion	Total Carbs (g)	Total Sugar (g)	Total Fat (g)	Recmmd.
Deep-filled apple pie	⅙ of 8 inch pie, 90 g (3 oz)	51	28	13	Avoid
Deep-filled blackcurrant pie	⅙ of 8 inch pie, 90 g (3 oz)	52	29	13	Avoid
Egg custard tart (individual)	1 tart	29	11	13	Avoid
Jam tart (individual)	1 tart	22	13	5	Avoid
Lemon meringue pie	⅙ of 7 inch pie, 75 g (2½ oz)	33	22	6	Avoid

DESSERTS (CONT.)

Food	Portion	Total Carbs (g)	Total Sugar (g)	Total Fat (g)	Recmmd.
Pastry, uncooked					
Filo	100 g (3½ oz)	60	1	4	Very Limited
Puff	100 g (3½ oz)	45	1	38	Avoid
Shortcrust	100 g (3½ oz)	47	1	28	Avoid
Treacle tart	⅛ of 8 inch tart, 75 g (2½ oz)	47	25	11	Avoid

PUDDINGS

Food	Portion	Total Carbs (g)	Total Sugar (g)	Total Fat (g)	Recmmd.
Bread pudding	100 g (3½ oz)	48	33	9	Avoid
Bread and butter pudding	125 g (4½ oz)	24	14	11	Avoid
Chocolate mousse, home-made	60 g (2 oz)	12	10	4	Avoid
Crème caramel	1 pot, 100 g (3½ oz)	21	18	2	Avoid
Custard sauces					
Crème anglaise/ egg custard, home-made	150 ml (¼ pt)	25	16	8	Avoid
Ready-made custard	150 ml (¼ pt)	24	19	4	Avoid
Custard, made w/semi-skimmed (low-fat) milk, from powder	150 ml (¼ pt)	25	17	3	Avoid

Food	Portion	Total Carbs (g)	Total Sugar (g)	Total Fat (g)	Recmmd.
Dessert, instant					
prepared w/semi-skimmed (low-fat) milk, chocolate	125 g (4½ oz)	15	12	4	Avoid
prepared w/semi-skimmed (low-fat) milk, strawberry	125 g (4½ oz)	14	11	4	Avoid
no added sugar, prepared w/skimmed milk, butterscotch	125 g (4½ oz)	11	5	2	Limited
ready-made chocolate (Weight Watchers)	1 pot, 100 g (3½ oz)	32	14	3	Avoid
Egg custard, baked	125 g (4½ oz)	20	13	10	Avoid
Fresh fruit salad	100 g (3½ oz)	15	14	Tr	Limited
Lemon mousse, light/low-fat	1 pot, 100 g (3½ oz)	17	16	2	Avoid
Pavlova, raspberry	1 slice, 60 g (2 oz)	25	24	8	Avoid
Raspberry mousse, light/low fat	1 pot, 100 g (3½ oz)	17	16	2	Avoid
Rice pudding					
canned, w/whole milk	200 g (7 oz)	32	17	3	Avoid
low-fat, canned	200 g (7 oz)	28	14	2	Avoid

DESSERTS (CONT.)

Food	Portion	Total Carbs (g)	Total Sugar (g)	Total Fat (g)	Recmmd.
Sticky toffee pudding	100 g (3½ oz)	47	34	12	Avoid
Summer pudding	100 g (3½ oz)	29	24	0.5	Avoid

DRINKS

Most fizzy drinks are very high in sugar: a can of cola contains 7 teaspoons of sugar. Diet drinks are OK in moderation, but water is the best choice for quenching thirst and hydrating your body.

Commercial fruit juices are often concentrates of the fruit's sugar without any of the fibre. You get much more nutritional benefit out of eating a whole fruit. If you need your glass of orange juice in the morning, fresh squeezed is best.

Both coffee and tea are major contributors of caffeine to our diets. Too much caffeine can cause a drop in blood sugar, leading to hunger and cravings. See pages 98–100 for milk and yogurt drinks.

Research suggests that moderate consumption of alcohol reduces the risk of heart disease and diabetes. We believe this is best accomplished by drinking red or white wine with meals. Beer is the worst choice because it contains maltose, the sugar with the highest glycaemic index. All alcohol is off-limits in Phase 1.

DRINKS, ALCOHOLIC

Food	Portion	Total Carbs (g)	Total Sugar (g)	Total Fat (g)	Recmmd.
Beers					
Bitter	300 ml (½ pt)	7	7	Tr	Avoid
Brown ale	300 ml (½ pt)	9	9	Tr	Avoid
Lager	300 ml (½ pt)	Tr	Tr	Tr	Avoid
Lager, low-alcohol	300 ml (½ pt)	4.5	3	0	Avoid

Food	Portion	Total Carbs (g)	Total Sugar (g)	Total Fat (g)	Recmmd.
Stout, sweet (e.g. Mackeson)	300 ml (½ pt)	6	6	Tr	Avoid
Stout, dry (e.g. Guinness)	300 ml (½ pt)	5	5	Tr	Avoid
Cider, dry	300 ml (½ pt)	8	8	0	Avoid
Cider, sweet	300 ml (½ pt)	13	13	0	Avoid
Liqueurs, clear	30 ml (1 fl oz)	11	11	0	Avoid
Liqueurs, creamy	30 ml (1 fl oz)	7	7	5	Avoid
Mixed drinks					
Rum and coke	135 ml (4½ fl oz)	11	11	0	Avoid
Mixed drinks in bottles (e.g. Bacardi Breezer)	275 ml (9 fl oz)	26	26	Tr	Avoid
Bloody Mary	135 ml (4½ fl oz)	3	3	Tr	Very Limited
Spirits (brandy, gin, rum, vodka, whisky)	30 ml (1 fl oz)	Tr	Tr	0	Allowed
Wines, dessert					
Madeira	60 ml (2 fl oz)	4	4	0	Avoid
Marsala	60 ml (2 fl oz)	4	4	0	Avoid
Port	60 ml (2 fl oz)	7	7	0	Avoid
Sherry	60 ml (2 fl oz)	4	4	0	Avoid
Wines, table					
Red	120 ml (4 fl oz)	Tr	Tr	0	Good
Rosé	120 ml (4 fl oz)	3	3	0	Good

DRINKS (CONT.)

Food	Portion	Total Carbs (g)	Total Sugar (g)	Total Fat (g)	Recmmd.
Dry white	120 ml (4 fl oz)	1	1	0	Good
Wine spritzer	300 ml (½ pt)	1	1	0	Good
Sparkling	120 ml (4 fl oz)	6	6	0	Good

DRINKS, NON-ALCOHOLIC

Food	Portion	Total Carbs (g)	Total Sugar (g)	Total Fat (g)	Recmmd.
Carbonated drinks					
Cola	330 ml (11 fl oz)	37	37	0	Avoid
Cola, diet	330 ml (11 fl oz)	Tr	Tr	0	Limited
Ginger ale	250 ml (8 fl oz)	10	10	0	Avoid
Ginger beer	330 ml (11 fl oz)	52	52	0	Avoid
Ginseng-type (e.g. Amé, Aqua Libra)	250 ml (8 fl oz)	12	12	0	Avoid
Lemon-lime (e.g. 7-up)	330 ml (11 fl oz)	35	35	0	Avoid
Lemonade	250 ml (8 fl oz)	15	15	0	Avoid
Lucozade	350 ml (12 fl oz)	60	53	0	Avoid
Orange	330 ml (11 fl oz)	35	35	Tr	Avoid
Soda water	250 ml (8 fl oz)	0	0	0	Allowed
Sparkling mineral water	250 ml (8 fl oz)	0	0	0	Good

Food	Portion	Total Carbs (g)	Total Sugar (g)	Total Fat (g)	Recmmd.
Tonic water	250 ml (8 fl oz)	22	22	0	Avoid
Tonic water, diet	250 ml (8 fl oz)	Tr	Tr	0	Limited
Sports drinks					
Lucozade Sport	500 ml (18 fl oz)	32	32	0	Avoid
Gatorade	330 ml (11 fl oz)	20	20	0	Avoid
Caffeinated drinks (e.g. Red Bull)	250 ml (8 fl oz)	28	28	0	Avoid
Protein shake (e.g. Slim-Fast)	325 ml can (11 fl oz)	34.5	34.5	2.5	Avoid
Coffee, brewed					
Black, regular	200 ml (7 fl oz)	0.5	0	Tr	Limited
Black, decaf	200 ml (7 fl oz)	0.5	0	Tr	Allowed
Black, w/1 tsp sugar	200 ml (7 fl oz)	5.5	5	Tr	Very Limited
w/2 tbsp single cream	200 ml (7 fl oz)	1	0.5	6	Very Limited
w/2 tbsp skimmed milk	200 ml (7 fl oz)	1	1	Tr	Limited
w/2 tbsp semi-skimmed (low-fat) milk	200 ml (7 fl oz)	2	1.5	0.5	Limited
w/2 tbsp whole milk	200 ml (7 fl oz)	2	1.5	1	Very Limited
w/1 tsp sugar and 2 tbsp whole milk	200 ml (7 fl oz)	7	6.5	1	Very Limited

DRINKS (CONT.)

Food	Portion	Total Carbs (g)	Total Sugar (g)	Total Fat (g)	Recmmd.
Coffee, espresso and cappuccino					
Cappuccino, w/milk, sugar and chocolate, takeaway	350 ml (12 fl oz)	30	30	3	Avoid
Cappuccino, w/milk, sugar and chocolate, restaurant	100 ml (3½ fl oz)	10	10	1	Avoid
Espresso	60 ml (2 fl oz)	0.5	0	Tr	Allowed
Latte, takeaway	350 ml (12 fl oz)	30	29	10	Avoid
Coffee, instant					
Instant, black	200 ml (7 fl oz)	0.5	0	Tr	Allowed
Instant, black w/1 tsp sugar	200 ml (7 fl oz)	5.5	5	Tr	Very Limited
Instant, black w/2 tbsp semi-skimmed (low-fat) milk	200 ml (7 fl oz)	2	1.5	0.5	Limited
Dairy drinks					
Chocolate flavoured drink, prepared w/skimmed milk, from mix	250 ml (8 fl oz)	25	22	2	Avoid
Chocolate flavoured soya drink	250 ml (8 fl oz)	25	22	5	Avoid

Food	Portion	Total Carbs (g)	Total Sugar (g)	Total Fat (g)	Recmmd.
Chocolate milk, low-fat	250 ml (8 fl oz)	50	44	4	Avoid
Hot chocolate, prepared w/whole milk, from powder	250 ml (8 fl oz)	28	28	11	Avoid
Milkshake, banana	250 ml (8 fl oz)	25	23	4	Avoid
Milkshake, chocolate	250 ml (8 fl oz)	25	22	4	Avoid
Milkshake, strawberry	250 ml (8 fl oz)	25	23	4	Avoid
Milkshake, vanilla	250 ml (8 fl oz)	25	22	4	Avoid
Milkshake, thickened type	500 ml (18 fl oz)	53	48	4	Avoid
Strawberry flavoured drink, prepared w/semi-skimmed (low-fat) milk, from mix	200 ml (7 fl oz)	20	19	3	Avoid
Vanilla flavoured sweetened soya drink	250 ml (8 fl oz)	28	24	6	Avoid
Teas					
Brewed tea, black	200 ml (7 fl oz)	Tr	Tr	Tr	Allowed
Brewed tea, black, w/1 tsp sugar	200 ml (7 fl oz)	5	5	Tr	Very Limited

DRINKS (CONT.)

Food	Portion	Total Carbs (g)	Total Sugar (g)	Total Fat (g)	Recmmd.
Brewed tea w/1 tbsp milk	200 ml (7 fl oz)	1	1	1	Allowed
Brewed tea, herbal	200 ml (7 fl oz)	Tr	Tr	Tr	Allowed
Iced tea, instant, sweetened w/sugar, prepared, w/water from mix	200 ml (7 fl oz)	14	14	Tr	Avoid
Iced tea, unsweetened/ diet, carton	250 ml (8 fl oz)	7	2	Tr	Allowed
Iced tea, ready-to-drink, fruit-flavoured, sweetened	250 ml (8 fl oz)	18	18	Tr	Avoid
Green tea	200 ml (7 fl oz)	Tr	Tr	Tr	Good

FRUIT DRINKS

Food	Portion	Total Carbs (g)	Total Sugar (g)	Total Fat (g)	Recmmd.
Juices					
Apple juice, unsweetened	200 ml (7 fl oz)	21	21	Tr	Very Limited
Apricot nectar	200 ml (7 fl oz)	29	29	Tr	Very Limited
Cranberry drink	200 ml (7 fl oz)	30	30	0	Avoid
Grape juice	200 ml (7 fl oz)	25	25	Tr	Very Limited

Food	Portion	Total Carbs (g)	Total Sugar (g)	Total Fat (g)	Recmmd.
Grapefruit juice, unsweetened	200 ml (7 fl oz)	17	17	Tr	Very Limited
Orange juice, freshly squeezed	200 ml (7 fl oz)	18	18	Tr	Very Limited
Orange juice, from concentrate	200 ml (7 fl oz)	18	18	Tr	Very Limited
Pineapple juice, unsweetened	200 ml (7 fl oz)	22	22	Tr	Very Limited
Prune juice, unsweetened	200 ml (7 fl oz)	32	28	Tr	Very Limited
Tomato juice, unsweetened	200 ml (7 fl oz)	6	6	Tr	Good
Tropical fruit blend	200 ml (7 fl oz)	25	25	Tr	Avoid
Vegetable juice (e.g. V8)	330 ml (11 fl oz)	17	17	Tr	Good
Smoothies					
Fruit (banana-based)	250 ml (8 fl oz)	35	32	0.5	Very Limited
Yogurt-based	250 ml (8 fl oz)	39	38	2	Very Limited
Juice-flavoured drinks, sweetened					
Blackcurrant and apple, carton	250 ml (8 fl oz)	26	26	Tr	Avoid
Mixed fruit drink, carton	250 ml (8 fl oz)	26	26	Tr	Avoid
Lemonade, homemade	250 ml (8 fl oz)	15	15	Tr	Avoid

DRINKS (CONT.)

Food	Portion	Total Carbs (g)	Total Sugar (g)	Total Fat (g)	Recmmd.
Orange juice drink, prepared w/water, from instant drink mix	250 ml (8 fl oz)	26	26	Tr	Avoid
Pouch-type	250 ml (8 fl oz)	26	26	Tr	Avoid
Squashes and cordials, diluted					
Blackcurrant cordial	250 ml (8 fl oz)	30	30	Tr	Avoid
High-juice squash	250 ml (8 fl oz)	25	25	Tr	Very Limited
Lime cordial	250 ml (8 fl oz)	27	27	Tr	Very Limited
Orange squash	250 ml (8 fl oz)	26	26	Tr	Avoid
Orange squash, no added sugar	250 ml (8 fl oz)	7	7	Tr	Limited

EGGS, EGG DISHES AND EGG SUBSTITUTES

The good news is that eggs are OK. They are rich in protein and the yolk is a good source of vitamin E. It is true that eggs are high in cholesterol, but they are also low in saturated fat. Eggs do increase cholesterol minimally, but they also increase HDL, the good cholesterol. Omelettes are a great way of including healthy vegetables in your breakfast, while hard-boiled eggs have the advantage of being fast and convenient.

EGGS, HENS'

Food	Portion	Total Carbs (g)	Total Sugar (g)	Total Fat (g)	Recmmd.
Extra large	1 each	Tr	Tr	8	Good

Food	Portion	Total Carbs (g)	Total Sugar (g)	Total Fat (g)	Recmmd.
Large	1 each	Tr	Tr	7	Good
Medium	1 each	Tr	Tr	6	Good
Small	1 each	Tr	Tr	5	Good
White only	1 extra-large	Tr	Tr	Tr	Good
Yolk only	1 extra-large	Tr	Tr	8	Good
Omega-3 fat enriched	1 large	Tr	Tr	6	Good

EGGS, OTHER

Food	Portion	Total Carbs (g)	Total Sugar (g)	Total Fat (g)	Recmmd.
Duck	1 large	1	Tr	10	Avoid
Quail	3 each	Tr	Tr	4	Good

EGG DISHES

Food	Portion	Total Carbs (g)	Total Sugar (g)	Total Fat (g)	Recmmd.
Boiled	1 large egg	Tr	Tr	6	Good
Fried, w/1 tsp butter	1 large egg	Tr	Tr	10	Limited
Fried, w/1 tsp trans-fat-free spread	1 serving	Tr	Tr	10	Good
Omelettes, 2-egg					
Plain, w/1 tsp trans-fat-free spread	1 serving	Tr	Tr	10	Good
Plain, w/2 tsp butter	1 serving	Tr	Tr	20	Limited

Food	Portion	Total Carbs (g)	Total Sugar (g)	Total Fat (g)	Recmmd.
w/30 g (1 oz) regular cheese	1 serving	Tr	Tr	22	Limited
w/30 g (1 oz) regular cheese + 30 g (1 oz) lean ham	1 serving	Tr	Tr	23	Limited
Pickled	1 large egg	Tr	Tr	7	Good
Poached	1 large egg	Tr	Tr	7	Good
Scrambled					
1 large egg, 1 tbsp milk + 1 tsp fat	1 large egg	0.5	0.5	12	Limited
1 large egg, 1 tbsp skimmed milk + no fat	1 serving	0.5	0.5	7	Good
2 large eggs, 2 tbsp milk + 2 tsp fat	1 serving	1	1	19	Limited
2 large eggs, 2 tbsp skimmed milk + no fat	1 serving	1	1	14	Good
Scotch egg	1 egg, 115 g (4 oz)	15	Tr	18	Avoid

EGG SUBSTITUTES

Food	Portion	Total Carbs (g)	Total Sugar (g)	Total Fat (g)	Recmmd.
Dried egg white	30 g (1 oz)	2	1	0	Good
Dried whole egg replacer	30 g (1 oz)	2	1	12	Good

FAST FOOD

Most fast foods fall into the 'avoid' category. They are dripping with saturated fats, trans fats, sugars and empty calories, and even the fish, chicken and veggie options at most fast-food outlets are coated with breadcrumbs and extra fat. But there are ways to eat wisely, even at a fast-food restaurant: choose grilled food instead of fried or deep-fried foods, and choose burgers without all the extra cheese and sauces. Ask for extra lettuce or tomato instead, or fill up at the salad bar. If pizza is your favourite fast food, turn to page 106.

When grabbing a sandwich, look for stoneground wholemeal, multigrain and seeded breads – and go easy on the mayonnaise.

BURGERS

Food	Portion	Total Carbs (g)	Total Sugar (g)	Total Fat (g)	Recmmd.
Cheeseburger, w/condiments, in a bun	1 burger, 125 g (4½ oz)	32	8	14	Avoid
Fish sandwich, breadcrumbed, w/tartare sauce	1	42	5	25	Avoid
Grilled chicken sandwich, breadcrumbed, w/mayonnaise	1	43	7	21	Avoid
Hamburger, quarter pounder w/condiments, in a bun	1 burger	34	8	24	Avoid
Hot dog, in a bun	1 bun, 145 g (5 oz)	36	2	14	Avoid
Nachos, w/cheese	145 g (5 oz)	72	2	35	Avoid
Veggieburger, w/condiments, in a bun	1 burger, 115 g (4 oz)	50	10	18	Avoid

FAST FOOD (CONT.)
SANDWICHES AND WRAPS

Food	Portion	Total Carbs (g)	Total Sugar (g)	Total Fat (g)	Recmmd.
Chicken fajita wrap	1 wrap 170 g (6 oz)	40	4	12	Avoid
Sandwiches					
BLT	170 g (6 oz)	41	4	22	Avoid
Chicken w/salad	170 g (6 oz)	40	4	14	Avoid
Cheese and pickle	170 g (6 oz)	48	7	25	Avoid
Egg mayonnaise	170 g (6 oz)	48	4	20	Avoid
Prawn mayonnaise	150 g (5½ oz)	43	4	19	Avoid
Roast beef w/horseradish	200 g (7 oz)	48	4	25	Avoid
Tuna and cucumber	170 g (6 oz)	40	4	20	Avoid
Vegetable tortilla wrap	1 wrap 200 g (7 oz)	41	4	20	Avoid

FAST FOOD CHICKEN

Food	Portion	Total Carbs (g)	Total Sugar (g)	Total Fat (g)	Recmmd.
Breast, crisp-fried	1 piece, 100 g (3½ oz)	15	1	13	Avoid
Chicken nuggets	6 pieces, 100 g (3½ oz)	11	Tr	15	Avoid
Drumstick, BBQ	1 piece, 100 g (3½ oz)	1	1	9	Avoid

Food	Portion	Total Carbs (g)	Total Sugar (g)	Total Fat (g)	Recmmd.
Drumstick, crisp-fried	1 piece, 75 g (2½ oz)	0	0	9	Avoid
Tandoori chicken fillets	100 g (3½ oz)	2	1	11	Avoid
Wings, Chinese style	1 serving 165 g	7	6	27	Avoid
Wings, hot and spicy	1 serving 165 g	7	5	27	Avoid

FAST FOOD POTATO ITEMS

Food	Portion	Total Carbs (g)	Total Sugar (g)	Total Fat (g)	Recmmd.
Baked potato, w/skin, plain	1 potato, 170 g (6 oz)	50	2	Tr	Avoid
Baked potato, w/skin, w/sour cream	1 potato, 170 g (6 oz)	51	3	6	Avoid
Baked potato, w/skin, w/tuna and sweetcorn	1 potato, 285 g (10 oz)	51	3	Tr	Avoid
Chips					
Oven, crinkle-cut	100 g (3½ oz)	30	0.5	5	Avoid
Deep-fried, medium-cut	100 g (3½ oz)	36	0.5	13	Avoid
Deep-fried, thin-cut	100 g (3½ oz)	41	0.5	21	Avoid

FATS AND OILS

With all the bad press fat has had over the last couple of decades, most people have concluded that simply limiting fats makes a diet healthy. This is a major mistake. While limiting saturated fat (meat- and dairy-derived) and avoiding trans fats (man-made hydrogenated and partially hydrogenated oils) as much as possible is important, there are other oils – including olive oil and omega-3 fish oils – that appear to be good for both our blood vessels and our waistlines. Nuts are also excellent sources of good fats and have been shown to help prevent heart attacks and strokes.

There is no advantage to low-fat diet dressings that substitute sugars and starches for healthy oils. Along with healthy oils, the vinegar in oil-and-vinegar dressings is acidic and helps slow digestion. This lowers the glycaemic index of the whole meal.

FATS

Food	Portion	Total Carbs (g)	Total Sugar (g)	Total Fat (g)	Recmmd.
Butter					
Half fat (40%)	1 tsp	Tr	Tr	2	Very Limited
	30 g (1 oz)	Tr	Tr	12	Avoid
Regular	1 tsp	Tr	Tr	4	Very Limited
	30 g (1 oz)	Tr	Tr	25	Avoid
Spreadable, reduced fat	1 tsp	Tr	Tr	3	Very Limited
	30 g (1 oz)	Tr	Tr	20	Avoid
Spreadable	1 tsp	Tr	Tr	4	Very Limited
	30 g (1 oz)	Tr	Tr	25	Avoid

Food	Portion	Total Carbs (g)	Total Sugar (g)	Total Fat (g)	Recmmd.
Ghee and other butters					
Ghee (clarified butter)	1 tbsp	Tr	Tr	11	Avoid
Ghee (clarified palm oil)	1 tbsp	Tr	Tr	11	Avoid
Ghee (vegetable oil)	1 tbsp	Tr	Tr	11	Avoid
Garlic butter	1 tbsp	Tr	Tr	9	Very Limited
Brandy butter	1 tbsp	4	4	7	Avoid
Margarine and spreads					
cholesterol-lowering (32% fat)	1 tsp	Tr	Tr	1.5	Good
cholesterol-lowering (63% fat)	1 tsp	Tr	Tr	3	Good
Cooking spray	2–3 second spray	0	0	0.5	Good
Trans-fat-free spread (e.g. I Can't Believe It's Not Butter!), regular	1 tsp	Tr	Tr	3	Good
Weight Watchers-type, light	1 tsp	Tr	Tr	1	Very Limited

FATS AND OILS (CONT.)

Food	Portion	Total Carbs (g)	Total Sugar (g)	Total Fat (g)	Recmmd.
Sunflower spread					
Light	1 tsp	Tr	Tr	2	Very Limited
Regular	1 tsp	Tr	Tr	4	Very Limited
Olive oil spread					
Light	1 tsp	Tr	Tr	2	Very Limited
Regular	1 tsp	Tr	Tr	3	Very Limited
Block margarine for cooking	30 g (1 oz)	Tr	Tr	24	Avoid
White fats					
Lard	30 g (1 oz)	0	0	30	Avoid
Beef dripping	30 g (1 oz)	Tr	Tr	30	Avoid
Vegetable fat	30 g (1 oz)	0	0	30	Avoid
Other fats					
Coconut cream, block	30 g (1 oz)	2	2	21	Avoid
Coconut milk, canned, unsweetened	100 ml (3½ fl oz)	3	3	20	Limited
Coconut, shredded, unsweetened	2 tbsp	2	2	18	Limited

OILS

Food	Portion	Total Carbs (g)	Total Sugar (g)	Total Fat (g)	Recmmd.
Avocado	1 tbsp	0	0	11	Good
Corn	1 tbsp	0	0	11	Limited
Grapeseed	1 tbsp	0	0	11	Limited
Olive	1 tbsp	0	0	11	Good
Olive, extra virgin	1 tbsp	0	0	11	Good
Palm	1 tbsp	0	0	11	Avoid
Peanut (groundnut)	1 tbsp	0	0	11	Good
Rapeseed (canola)	1 tbsp	0	0	11	Good
Safflower	1 tbsp	0	0	11	Limited
Sesame	1 tbsp	0	0	11	Limited
Soya	1 tbsp	0	0	11	Limited
Sunflower	1 tbsp	0	0	11	Limited
Vegetable	1 tbsp	0	0	11	Limited
Walnut	1 tbsp	0	0	11	Good

FISH AND SHELLFISH

All fish is low in saturated fat, and many varieties of fish contain a good type of fat called omega-3. Omega-3, found in fish oil, appears to benefit us in several ways. As well as helping prevent heart attacks and strokes, there is evidence that fish oil helps prevent or treat depression, arthritis, asthma and dry skin. It may also help us lose weight.

Shellfish, such as prawns, were once labelled high in cholesterol, and avoided by people with concerns about their diets. But this has been proven wrong. Feel free to enjoy all shellfish on the South Beach Diet. However, the mercury content of fish is a growing concern. Canned tuna and swordfish should be limited for this reason.

FISH, BAKED OR GRILLED

Food	Portion	Total Carbs (g)	Total Sugar (g)	Total Fat (g)	Recmmd.
Barramundi	100 g (3½ oz)	0	0	1	Good
Bass, sea	100 g (3½ oz)	0	0	1	Good
Bream, sea	100 g (3½ oz)	0	0	1	Good
Cod, dried, salted, boiled	100 g (3½ oz)	0	0	1	Good
Cod fillet	100 g (3½ oz)	0	0	1	Good
Haddock fillet	100 g (3½ oz)	0	0	1	Good
Haddock, smoked	100 g (3½ oz)	0	0	1	Good
Hake steak	100 g (3½ oz)	0	0	1	Good
Halibut	100 g (3½ oz)	0	0	2	Good
Herring, filleted	100 g (3½ oz)	0	0	13	Good
Herring, pickled	100 g (3½ oz)	7	1	18	Good
Hoki fillet	100 g (3½ oz)	0	0	1	Good
John Dory	100 g (3½ oz)	0	0	2	Good
Kabeljou	100 g (3½ oz)	0	0	2	Good
Kingklip	100 g (3½ oz)	0	0	1	Good

Food	Portion	Total Carbs (g)	Total Sugar (g)	Total Fat (g)	Recmmd.
Kipper, whole	170 g (6 oz)	0	0	30	Good
Kipper fillets	100 g (3½ oz)	0	0	18	Good
Mackerel	100 g (3½ oz)	0	0	16	Good
Monkfish	100 g (3½ oz)	0	0	2	Good
Perch	100 g (3½ oz)	0	0	2	Good
Plaice	100 g (3½ oz)	0	0	1	Good
Salmon					
Fresh	100 g (3½ oz)	0	0	11	Good
Gravadlax	50 g (1¾ oz)	0	0	4	Good
Smoked	50 g (1¾ oz)	0	0	4	Good
Sardines (6)	100 g (3½ oz)	0	0	10	Good
Skate wing	100 g (3½ oz)	0	0	2	
Snapper, red	100 g (3½ oz)	0	0	2	Good
Snoek	100 g (3½ oz)	0	0	12	Good
Sole, Dover whole w/bone	250 g (9 oz)	0	0	4	Good
Sole, lemon	100 g (3½ oz)	0	0	1	Good
Squid	100 g (3½ oz)	0	Tr	2	Good
Swordfish	100 g (3½ oz)	0	0	5	Good
Trout, rainbow	100 g (3½ oz)	0	0	5	Good
Trout, sea	100 g (3½ oz)	0	0	5	Good
Tuna, fresh	100 g (3½ oz)	0	0	1	Good
Whitebait, floured and fried	100 g (3½ oz)	5	Tr	47	Avoid
Whiting	100 g (3½ oz)	0	0	2	Good

FISH AND SHELLFISH (CONT.)
FISH, CRUMBED OR IN BATTER

Food	Portion	Total Carbs (g)	Total Sugar (g)	Total Fat (g)	Recmmd.
Calamari/squid rings	150 g (5½ oz)	23	3	15	Avoid
Cod fishcakes	2, 100 g (3½ oz)	17	Tr	13	Avoid
Fish and chips	250 g (9 oz)	47	2	35	Avoid
Fish fillet in crispy batter	125 g (4½ oz)	15	Tr	19	Avoid
Fish fillet, crumbed, oven baked	100 g (3½ oz)	14	2	8	Avoid
Fish fingers, crumbed, oven baked	100 g (3½ oz)	17	Tr	9	Avoid
Fish fingers in batter	100 g (3½ oz)	16	2	12	Avoid
Salmon fishcakes	2, 100 g (3½ oz)	17	1	7	Avoid
Scampi in breadcrumbs, fried	170 g (6 oz)	35	Tr	23	Avoid

FISH, CANNED

Food	Portion	Total Carbs (g)	Total Sugar (g)	Total Fat (g)	Recmmd.
Anchovies, in oil, drained	5, 15 g (½ oz)	0	0	2	Good
Pilchards in tomato sauce	100 g (3½ oz)	1	1	8	Good

Food	Portion	Total Carbs (g)	Total Sugar (g)	Total Fat (g)	Recmmd.
Mackerel in tomato sauce	125 g (4½ oz)	2	1.5	11	Good
Salmon, pink or red, drained	125 g (4½ oz)	0	0	8	Good
Sardines					
in oil, drained	90 g (3 oz)	0	0	13	Good
in tomato sauce	120 g (4½ oz)	2	2	12	Good
in brine. drained	90 g (3 oz)	0	0	9	Good
Tuna					
Chunks, in oil, drained	90 g (3 oz)	0	0	8	Good
Chunks, in brine or water, drained	90 g (3 oz)	0	0	0.5	Good
Steak, in oil, drained	90 g (3 oz)	0	0	8	Good
Steak, in brine or water, drained	90 g (3 oz)	0	0	0.5	Good

FISH, ROE AND EGGS

Food	Portion	Total Carbs (g)	Total Sugar (g)	Total Fat (g)	Recmmd.
Herring roe, soft	100 g (3½ oz)	Tr	Tr	4	Good
Salmon roe (keta)	30 g (1 oz)	Tr	Tr	4	Good
Lumpfish roe	30 g (1 oz)	2	0	4	Good
Cod roe, firm	50 g (1¾ oz)	3	0	4	Good

FISH AND SHELLFISH (CONT.)
SHELLFISH

Food	Portion	Total Carbs (g)	Total Sugar (g)	Total Fat (g)	Recmmd.
Clams	100 g (3½ oz)	Tr	Tr	0.5	Good
Crab					
Canned	100 g (3½ oz)	Tr	Tr	0.5	Good
Dressed	145 g (5 oz)	Tr	Tr	8	Limited
Fresh	100 g (3½ oz)	Tr	Tr	6	Good
Crabstick	1, 15 g (½ oz)	1	Tr	Tr	Good
Crayfish	100 g (3½ oz)	Tr	Tr	2	Good
Lobster, meat only	100 g (3½ oz)	Tr	Tr	2	Good
Mussels, flesh only	100 g (3½ oz)	Tr	Tr	3	Good
Oysters, shelled	6, 90 g (3 oz)	Tr	Tr	3	Good
Prawns, shelled	100 g (3½ oz)	0	0	1	Good
Scallops	100 g (3½ oz)	1	Tr	Tr	Good
Shrimps, potted	100 g (3½ oz)	Tr	Tr	1	Good

SUSHI

Food	Portion	Total Carbs (g)	Total Sugar (g)	Total Fat (g)	Recmmd.
Nori roll/maki	15 g (½ oz)	5	1	Tr	Avoid
Raw fish on rice/ nigiri	30 g (1 oz)	7	2	1	Avoid

FRUIT

Because of their carbohydrate, fibre, vitamin and mineral content, most fruit can be eaten frequently after Phase 1. Some fruits are high in sugar and should be eaten in limited amounts. We encourage the consumption of whole fruit. Avoid canned fruits packed in heavy syrup and processed commercial fruit juices.

FRUIT, CANNED

Food	Portion	Total Carbs (g)	Total Sugar (g)	Total Fat (g)	Recmmd.
Apricots, in juice	115 g (4 oz)	10	10	0	Very Limited
Cherries, in syrup	100 g (3½ oz)	18	18	Tr	Avoid
Fruit cocktail, in juice	115 g (4 oz)	8	8	Tr	Very Limited
Grapefruit, in juice	115 g (4 oz)	8	8	Tr	Very Limited
Mandarin oranges, in juice	115 g (4 oz)	9	9	Tr	Very Limited
Peaches					
in juice	115 g (4 oz)	11	11	Tr	Very Limited
in light syrup	115 g (4 oz)	16	16	Tr	Very Limited
Pear halves					
in juice	115 g (4 oz)	10	10	Tr	Very Limited
in syrup	115 g (4 oz)	15	15	Tr	Very Limited
Pineapple					
pieces, in juice	115 g (4 oz)	14	14	Tr	Very Limited

FRUIT, CANNED (CONT.)

Food	Portion	Total Carbs (g)	Total Sugar (g)	Total Fat (g)	Recmmd.
chunks, in light syrup	115 g (4 oz)	19	19	Tr	Avoid
Prunes, in juice	115 g (4 oz)	23	23	Tr	Very Limited

FRUIT, DRIED

Food	Portion	Total Carbs (g)	Total Sugar (g)	Total Fat (g)	Recmmd.
Apple rings	30 g (1 oz)	12	12	Tr	Good
Apricots, ready to eat	30 g (1 oz)	11	11	Tr	Good
Apricots	30 g (1 oz)	12	12	Tr	Good
Cherries	30 g (1 oz)	22	21	0.5	Very Limited
Cranberries	30 g (1 oz)	23	20	0.5	Very Limited
Coconut, desiccated, unsweetened	30 g (1 oz)	2	2	19	Very Limited
Currants	30 g (1 oz)	20	20	Tr	Avoid
Dates, pitted	30 g (1 oz)	20	20	Tr	Avoid
Figs	30 g (1 oz)	15	15	0.5	Avoid
Mango	30 g (1 oz)	10	10	0	Very Limited
Prunes, pitted	30 g (1 oz)	10	10	Tr	Good
Raisins	30 g (1 oz)	21	21	Tr	Very Limited
Sultanas	30 g (1 oz)	21	21	Tr	Avoid

FRUIT, FRESH

Food	Portion	Total Carbs (g)	Total Sugar (g)	Total Fat (g)	Recmmd.
Apple	1 medium, 100 g (3½ oz)	12	12	Tr	Good
Apricots	3, 125 g (4½ oz)		9	Tr	Good
Banana, ripe	1 medium, 150 g (5½ oz)	35	31	0.5	Limited
Blueberries	100 g (3½ oz)	5	5	Tr	Good
Blackberries, raw	100 g (3½ oz)	5	5	Tr	Good
Blackcurrants, stewed without sugar	100 g (3½ oz)	6	6	Tr	Good
Cherries, pitted	100 g (3½ oz)	11	11	Tr	Limited
Cranberries	100 g (3½ oz)	5	5	Tr	Good
Dates, fresh	3, 90 g (3 oz)	28	28	Tr	Limited
Fig	1, 40 g (1¼ oz)	10	10	0.5	Good
Gooseberries	100 g (3½ oz)	3	3	Tr	Good
Grapefruit	½, 170 g (6 oz)	11	11	Tr	Good
Grapes, red or green	20 grapes, 100 g (3½ oz)	15	15	Tr	Good
Guava	1, 90 g (3 oz)	5	5	0.5	Good
Kiwi fruit	1, 60 g (2 oz)	7	7	Tr	Good
Lemon	1 slice	Tr	Tr	Tr	Good
Lime	75 g (2½ oz)	2	2	Tr	Good
Lychees	100 g (3½ oz)	14	14	Tr	Good
Mango	100 g (3½ oz)	14	14	Tr	Limited

FRUIT, FRESH (CONT.)

Food	Portion	Total Carbs (g)	Total Sugar (g)	Total Fat (g)	Recmmd.
Melon					
Green-fleshed	100 g (3½ oz)	6	6	Tr	Limited
Honeydew	100 g (3½ oz)	7	7	Tr	Limited
Orange-fleshed	100 g (3½ oz)	4	4	Tr	Limited
Watermelon	100 g (3½ oz)	7	7	Tr	Avoid
Nectarine	1 medium, 145 g (5 oz)	13	13	Tr	Good
Orange	1 medium, 145 g (5 oz)	12	12	Tr	Good
Papaya/paw paw	1 small, 230 g (8 oz)	20	20	Tr	Limited
Passion fruit	1, 15 g (½ oz)	1	1	Tr	Good
Peach	1 medium, 115 g (4 oz)	9	9	Tr	Good
Pear	1 medium, 145 g (5 oz)	14	14	Tr	Good
Pineapple	250 g (9 oz)	25	25	0.5	Very Limited
Plum	2 small	13	13	Tr	Good
Prickly pear	1 medium, 100 g (3½ oz)	10	7	0.5	Good
Raspberries	100 g (3½ oz)	5	5	Tr	Good
Rhubarb, stewed with sugar	100 g (3½ oz)	11	11	Tr	Very Limited
Strawberries	100 g (3½ oz)	6	6	Tr	Good
Tangerine, satsuma, mandarin, clementine	1 medium, 75 g (2½ oz)	6	6	Tr	Good

GRAINS AND RICE

Enjoy grains frequently, as long as you eat the right ones. The more intact the grain, the higher the fibre and nutrition. Whole grains, including wheat, rye, barley, corn, and some types of rice, are rich in bran, B vitamins, iron and other minerals. Stay away from white rice, which has been milled, removing many of the nutrients. Brown rice is a much better source of B vitamins, minerals and fibre. Wild rice is frequently served in combination with white or brown rice and is very nutritious and low on the glycaemic index. Couscous is another good low-glycaemic index choice to substitute for white rice or white potatoes.

GRAINS

Food	Portion	Total Carbs (g)	Total Sugar (g)	Total Fat (g)	Recmmd.
Arrowroot	1 tbsp	18	Tr	Tr	Limited
Barley, pearl, boiled	100 g (3½ oz)	28	Tr	Tr	Good
Buckwheat (kasha), cooked	50 g (1¾ oz)	10	0.5	0.5	Good
Bulgur wheat, cooked	100 g (3½ oz)	18	Tr	Tr	Good
Cornflour	1 tbsp	28	Tr	Tr	Very Limited
Cornmeal/ polenta, cooked	100 g (3½ oz) from 30 g (1 oz) raw	19	Tr	Tr	Limited
Couscous	75 g (2½ oz)	19	2	1	Limited
Millet grain	75 g (2½ oz)	18	Tr	Tr	Avoid
Oatmeal, cooked	100 g (3½ oz)	11	1.5	1	Good
Rye, whole kernel	75 g (2½ oz)	20	Tr	1	Good
Semolina, cooked	100 g (3½ oz)	24	Tr	Tr	Limited
Wheatgerm	1 tbsp	5	2	1	Good

GRAINS AND RICE (CONT.)
RICE, COOKED

Food	Portion	Total Carbs (g)	Total Sugar (g)	Total Fat (g)	Recmmd.
Basmati	170 g (6 oz)	49	Tr	0.5	Limited
Brown	170 g (6 oz)	54	1	2	Good
Brown, quick-cooking	170 g (6 oz)	55	1	2	Avoid
Camargue red rice	170 g (6 oz)	32	1	1	Good
Glutinous	170 g (6 oz)	51	Tr	2	Avoid
Jasmine	170 g (6 oz)	51	Tr	2	Avoid
Ground rice	100 g (3½ oz)	30	Tr	1	Avoid
Risotto rice	170 g (6 oz)	48	Tr	1	Avoid
Pudding, made with milk and sugar	170 g (6 oz)	33	18	7	Avoid
White, quick-cooking	170 g (6 oz)	53	Tr	2	Avoid
White, long-grain	170 g (6 oz)	50	Tr	2	Limited
White, easy-cook	170 g (6 oz)	53	Tr	2	Avoid
Wild	170 g (6 oz)	47	1	3	Good

ICE CREAM AND FROZEN DESSERTS

Ice cream is not a part of the South Beach Diet, although you can enjoy a small amount as a *very* occasional treat. Look for lower-fat options such as sorbet and frozen yogurt (though they're still high in sugar) or sugar-free ice pops.

ICE CREAM

Food	Portion	Total Carbs (g)	Total Sugar (g)	Total Fat (g)	Recmmd.
Low-fat					
Chocolate, Weight Watchers	100 ml (3½ fl oz)	12	12	1.5	Very Limited
Vanilla (95% fat-free)	100 ml (3½ fl oz)	12	11	1.5	Very Limited
Premium					
Cookies and cream	100 ml (3½ fl oz)	20	18	14	Avoid
Cornish vanilla	100 ml (3½ fl oz)	11	11	10	Avoid
Maple and walnut	100 ml (3½ fl oz)	20	18	14	Avoid
Mint chocolate chip	100 ml (3½ fl oz)	19	17	13	Avoid
Regular					
Chocolate	100 ml (3½ fl oz)	11	11	3.5	Very Limited
Raspberry ripple	100 ml (3½ fl oz)	11	11	3.5	Very Limited
Strawberry	100 ml (3½ fl oz)	11	10	3.4	Very Limited
Vanilla	100 ml (3½ fl oz)	8	8	2.5	Very Limited

ICE CREAM BARS, CONES AND LOLLIES

Food	Portion	Total Carbs (g)	Total Sugar (g)	Total Fat (g)	Recmmd.
Blackcurrant lolly (ice block)	50 g (1¾ oz)	9	8	Tr	Limited

ICE CREAMS (CONT.)

Food	Portion	Total Carbs (g)	Total Sugar (g)	Total Fat (g)	Recmmd.
Choc ice	60 g (2 oz)	14	12	13	Avoid
Chocolate and vanilla cone	75 g (2½ oz)	22	14	13	Avoid
Chocolate mini lolly	30 g (1 oz)	10	8	5	Avoid
Whipped ice cream cone	125 ml (4 fl oz)	8	8	3	Avoid
Orange juice lolly (ice block)	75 g (2½ oz)	14	13	Tr	Limited
Luxury chocolate-coated ice cream (e.g. Magnum)	75 g (2½ oz)	16	15	17	Avoid
Sugar-free ice pops	20 ml	Tr	Tr	Tr	Allowed

FROZEN DESSERTS

Food	Portion	Total Carbs (g)	Total Sugar (g)	Total Fat (g)	Recmmd.
Frozen yoghurt	100 ml (3½ fl oz)	9	9	1	Limited
Sorbet					
Lemon	100 ml (3½ fl oz)	19	18	Tr	Very Limited
Mango	100 ml (3½ fl oz)	19	19	Tr	Very Limited
Raspberry	100 ml (3½ fl oz)	24	23	Tr	Very Limited
Tofu-based, frozen dessert	100 ml (3½ fl oz)	23	22	13	Very Limited
Viennetta, vanilla	75 g (2½ oz)	16	15	13	Avoid

Many cuts of beef are appropriate for a heart-healthy diet; lean pork and lamb may be enjoyed occasionally, too.

Processed meats include the many types of hot and cold sausage, pâté and cold cuts. Most of these products contain sodium nitrate as a preservative for longer shelf life and are, as a rule, high in saturated fat and sodium.

Tofu, tempeh and other soya-based foods are all good meat substitutes. When you eat these, you also benefit from soya's cholesterol-lowering properties.

BEEF

Food	Portion	Total Carbs (g)	Total Sugar (g)	Total Fat (g)	Recmmd.
Beef roasts					
Topside	100 g (3½ oz)	0	0	5	Good
Sirloin	100 g (3½ oz)	0	0	5	Good
Rolled rib	100 g (3½ oz)	0	0	10	Limited
Forerib w/bone	100 g (3½ oz)	0	0	10	Limited
Stewing/ braising					
Braising steak	100 g (3½ oz)	0	0	8	Limited
Salt beef (brisket)	100 g (3½ oz)	0	0	6	Limited
Shin	100 g (3½ oz)	0	0	6	Limited
Silverside	100 g (3½ oz)	0	0	5	Good
Stewing steak (chuck)	100 g (3½ oz)	0	0	6	Limited
Steaks					
Rib eye	230 g (8 oz)	0	0	5	Limited
Fillet	150 g (5 oz)	0	0	5	Good
Sirloin	230 g (8 oz)	0	0	5	Good

MEAT (CONT.)

Food	Portion	Total Carbs (g)	Total Sugar (g)	Total Fat (g)	Recmmd.
Rump	230 g (8 oz)	0	0	5	Good
T-bone	230 g (8 oz)	0	0	5	Good
Minced beef					
Extra lean (5% fat)	100 g (3½ oz)	0	0	5	Good
Lean (less than 10% fat)	100 g (3½ oz)	0	0	9	Limited
Regular (15% fat)	100 g (3½ oz)	0	0	15	Very Limited

LAMB, LEAN

Food	Portion	Total Carbs (g)	Total Sugar (g)	Total Fat (g)	Recmmd.
Chump chop	125 g (4½ oz)	0	0	11	Limited
Crown roast or rack	100 g (3½ oz)	0	0	15	Limited
Cutlet	100 g (3½ oz)	0	0	12	Limited
Leg of lamb					
Leg, shank end	100 g (3½ oz)	0	0	8	Limited
Leg, fillet end	100 g (3½ oz)	0	0	8	Limited
Whole leg	100 g (3½ oz)	0	0	10	Limited
Loin	100g (3½ oz)	0	0	10	Limited
Minced lamb (20% fat)	100 g (3½ oz)	0	0	20	Avoid
Shoulder	100 g (3½ oz)	0	0	11	Limited
Stewing lamb, cubed	170 g (6 oz)	0	0	23	Avoid

PORK

Food	Portion	Total Carbs (g)	Total Sugar (g)	Total Fat (g)	Recmmd.
Pork roasts					
Leg	100 g (3½ oz)	0	0	5	Good
Loin, w/bone	100 g (3½ oz)	0	0	6	Good
Rolled loin	100 g (3½ oz)	0	0	20	Avoid
Leg fillet, w/bone	100 g (3½ oz)	0	0	4	Good
Pork chops and steaks					
Loin chop, w/kidney	170 g (6 oz)	0	0	8	Limited
Loin chop	150 g (5½ oz)	0	0	9	Limited
Shoulder chop/ spare rib chop	100 g (3½ oz)	0	0	8	Limited
Pork fillet or tenderloin	100 g (3½ oz)	0	0	6	Good
Spare rib rack	170 g (6 oz)	0	0	23	Avoid
Other cuts					
Belly	150 g (5½ oz)	0	0	25	Avoid
Minced pork	100 g (3½ oz)	0	0	14	Avoid

PORK, CURED

Food	Portion	Total Carbs (g)	Total Sugar (g)	Total Fat (g)	Recmmd.
Back rasher	30 g (1 oz)	0	0	2	Good
Collar	100 g (3½ oz)	0	0	10	Avoid
Hock	100 g (3½ oz)	0	0	10	Avoid
Pancetta	30 g (1 oz)	0	0	8	Limited

MEAT (CONT.)

Food	Portion	Total Carbs (g)	Total Sugar (g)	Total Fat (g)	Recmmd.
Streaky rasher	2 rashers 40 g (1¼ oz)	0	0	9	Avoid
Ham, cured, boiled or roasted					
Boneless, extra-lean	40 g (1¼ oz)	0	0	1	Good
Boneless, lean	40 g (1¼ oz)	0	0	1	Good
Canned, extra-lean	40 g (1¼ oz)	0	0	1	Good
Gammon steak	125 g (4½ oz)	0	0	9	Limited
Gammon joint	100 g (3½ oz)	0	0	7	Limited

VEAL, LEAN

Food	Portion	Total Carbs (g)	Total Sugar (g)	Total Fat (g)	Recmmd.
Cutlet, w/bone	150 g (5½ oz)	0	0	3	Good
Escalope	150 g (5½ oz)	0	0	4	Good
Loin, boned and rolled	100 g (3½ oz)	0	0	3	Good
Minced veal	150 g (5½ oz)	0	0	4	Good
Osso bucco	340 g (12 oz)	8	6	15	Avoid
Stewing veal	150 g (5½ oz)	0	0	4	Good

OFFAL

Food	Portion	Total Carbs (g)	Total Sugar (g)	Total Fat (g)	Recmmd.
Ox kidney	30 g (1 oz)	0	0	1	Avoid
Ox heart	100 g (3½ oz)	0	0	12	Avoid

Food	Portion	Total Carbs (g)	Total Sugar (g)	Total Fat (g)	Recmmd.
Ox tongue	100 g (3½ oz)	0	0	20	Avoid
Oxtail	170 g (6 oz)	0	0	22	Avoid
Lambs' kidneys	1 kidney 40 g (1¼ oz)	0	0	2	Avoid
Lambs' liver	40 g (1¼ oz)	Tr	0	3	Avoid
Pigs' kidneys	1 kidney 40 g (1¼ oz)	0	0	2	Avoid
Pigs' liver	50 g (1¾ oz)	2	0	4	Avoid
Calves' liver	100 g (3½ oz)	Tr	0	7	Avoid
Lambs' hearts	170 g (6 oz)	0	0	20	Avoid
Sweetbreads	100 g (3½ oz)	0	0	9	Avoid
Tripe	100 g (3½ oz)	0	0	0.5	Avoid

PROCESSED MEATS

Food	Portion	Total Carbs (g)	Total Sugar (g)	Total Fat (g)	Recmmd.
Cold cuts					
Chicken roll	60 g (2 oz)	3	0	3	Limited
Corned beef	60 g (2 oz)	0.5	0.5	7	Limited
Biltong	30 g (1 oz)	Tr	Tr	2	Limited
Bresaola	60 g (2 oz)	Tr	Tr	3	Limited
Garlic sausage	60 g (2 oz)	2	1	7	Avoid
Ham, wafer thin	60 g (2 oz)	0.5	0.5	2	Good
Ham, honey roast	60 g (2 oz)	0.5	0.5	2	Limited
Ham, dry-cured (e.g. Parma)	60 g (2 oz)	Tr	Tr	8	Limited
Ham, turkey	60 g (2 oz)	0.5	0.5	2	Good

PROCESSED MEATS (CONT.)

Food	Portion	Total Carbs (g)	Total Sugar (g)	Total Fat (g)	Recmmd.
Liver sausage	60 g (2 oz)	4	0.5	10	Avoid
Mortadella	60 g (2 oz)	0	0	17	Avoid
Pastrami, beef	60 g (2 oz)	1	1	3	Avoid
Pastrami, turkey	60 g (2 oz)	1	1	3	Good
Pâté	60 g (2 oz)	0.5	Tr	18	Avoid
Pork luncheon meat	60 g (2 oz)	2	Tr	14	Avoid
Salami	60 g (2 oz)	0.5	0.5	18	Avoid
Salami, peppered	60 g (2 oz)	0.5	0.5	18	Avoid
Turkey bacon	2 rashers, 50 g (1¾ oz)	1.5	1.5	1	Good
Turkey breast, smoked	60 g (2 oz)	0	0	1	Good
Turkey salami	60 g (2 oz)	11	4	5	Limited
Sausages, cooked					
Bockwurst	50 g (1¾ oz)	1	1	12	Avoid
Black pudding	50 g (1¾ oz)	8	Tr	10	Avoid
Bratwurst	50 g (1¾ oz)	1	1	11	Avoid
Chorizo	50 g (1¾ oz)	1	1	12	Avoid
Frankfurters, canned	1, 30 g (1 oz)	1	Tr	3	Avoid
Frankfurter, American style	1, 50 g (1¾ oz)	2	Tr	12	Avoid
Merguez	50 g (1¾ oz)	1	1	15	Avoid
Pork, 65% meat	50 g (1¾ oz)	5	1.5	12	Avoid

Food	Portion	Total Carbs (g)	Total Sugar (g)	Total Fat (g)	Recmmd.
Pork, 95% meat	50 g (1¾ oz)	3	0.5	10	Avoid
Pork, low-fat	50 g (1¾ oz)	5	0.5	7	Avoid
Pork and beef	50 g (1¾ oz)	5	1	11	Avoid
Turkey hot dog	1, 45 g (1½ oz)	Tr	0	7	Limited
Turkey sausage	50 g (1¾ oz)	3	1	5	Limited

MEAT SUBSTITUTES

Food	Portion	Total Carbs (g)	Total Sugar (g)	Total Fat (g)	Recmmd.
Burgers and sausages					
Spicy bean burger	1, 100 g (3½ oz)	8	4	11	Limited
Meat-free hot dog	1, 30 g (1 oz)	3	2	2	Good
Vegetable and tofu burger	1, 100 g (3½ oz)	7	1	8	Good
Vegeburger	1, 60 g (2 oz)	5	2	7	Good
Vegetarian sausage (soya)	1, 50 g (1¾ oz)	4	0.5	5	Good
Quorn chunks	100 g (3½ oz)	6	1.5	3	Good
Quorn burger	1 burger, 50 g (1¾ oz)	4	1	2	Good
Quorn sausages	1 sausage, 35 g (1¼ oz)	2	Tr	1	Good
Quorn bacon	1 'rasher', 30 g (1½ oz)	2	Tr	1.5	Good
Soya mince (TVP), reconstituted	100 g (3½ oz)	20	4	3	Good
Tempeh	50 g (1¾ oz)	3	2	3	Good

MEAT SUBSTITUTES (CONT.)

Food	Portion	Total Carbs (g)	Total Sugar (g)	Total Fat (g)	Recmmd.
Tofu (bean curd)					
Marinated pieces	50 g (1¾ oz)	0.5	Tr	3	Good
Natural	50 g (1¾ oz)	0.5	Tr	3	Good
Smoked	50 g (1¾ oz)	0.5	Tr	3	Good

MILK, MILK PRODUCTS AND MILK SUBSTITUTES

Dairy products are an excellent source of calcium and protein and make great snacks. But whole-milk dairy products, such as butter, cheese, milk, cream and ice cream, contain high amounts of saturated fat. When selecting dairy products, look for skimmed or semi-skimmed (low-fat) milk, reduced-fat cheese, and low-fat or fat-free natural yogurt. These products contain the milk sugar lactose, which has a moderate glycaemic index, lower than other simple sugars. Also look for low-fat soya milk and soya drinks, which contain more protein and less fat than cow's milk.

CREAMS AND CREAM SUBSTITUTES

Food	Portion	Total Carbs (g)	Total Sugar (g)	Total Fat (g)	Recmmd.
Cream					
Single/pouring (19% fat)	1 tbsp	Tr	Tr	3	Avoid
Whipping (39% fat)	1 tbsp	Tr	Tr	6	Avoid
Double (48% fat)	1 tbsp	Tr	Tr	8	Avoid
Clotted	1 tbsp	Tr	Tr	10	Avoid
Sour	1 tbsp	0.5	0.5	3	Limited
Sour, extra light	1 tbsp	1	1	2	Limited

Food	Portion	Total Carbs (g)	Total Sugar (g)	Total Fat (g)	Recmmd.
Aerosol	30 ml (1 fl oz)	2	2	7	Very Limited
Crème fraîche	1 tbsp	Tr	Tr	6	Avoid
Crème fraîche, half fat	1 tbsp	0.5	0.5	3	Very Limited
Extra thick	1 tbsp	Tr	Tr	10	Avoid
Canned	1 tbsp	0.5	0.5	4	Avoid
UHT single	1 tbsp	Tr	Tr	3	Avoid
UHT double	1 tbsp	Tr	Tr	8	Avoid
UHT, reduced-fat, sweetened	1 tbsp	1	1	2	Very Limited
Coffee whitener powder	1 tsp	2	2	1	Limited
Soya 'cream' (e.g. Provamel Soya Dream)	1 tbsp	Tr	Tr	3	Limited
Toppings					
Dessert topping made from powder (e.g. Dream Topping)	2 tbsp	4	3	4	Avoid
Dessert topping, sugar-free	2 tbsp	3	1	3	Very Limited
Cream alternative (e.g. Elmlea)					
Single	1 tbsp	0.5	0.5	2	Limited
Double	1 tbsp	0.5	0.5	5	Avoid
Light	1 tbsp	0.5	0.5	1	Limited

MILK, MILK PRODUCTS AND MILK SUBSTITUTES (CONT.)
FROMAGE FRAIS

Food	Portion	Total Carbs (g)	Total Sugar (g)	Total Fat (g)	Recmmd.
Fromage frais, natural	100 g (3½ oz)	4	4	8	Limited
Fromage frais virtually fat-free	100 g (3½ oz)	5	4	Tr	Good
Fromage frais with fruit, sweetened	100 g (3½ oz)	14	13	6	Avoid

MILK AND NON-DAIRY MILKS

Food	Portion	Total Carbs (g)	Total Sugar (g)	Total Fat (g)	Recmmd.
Buttermilk	150 ml (5 fl oz)	9	8	Tr	Good
Chocolate milk					
Low-fat	200 ml (7 fl oz)	18	16	3	Very Limited
Whole milk, thickened	200 ml (7 fl oz)	30	22	8	Avoid
Cow's milk					
Skimmed	250 ml (8 fl oz)	11	11	0.5	Good
Semi-skimmed (low-fat)	250 ml (8 fl oz)	12	12	4	Very Limited
Whole	250 ml (8 fl oz)	11	11	10	Avoid
Longlife/UHT skimmed	250 ml (8 fl oz)	10	10	0.5	Good
Longlife/UHT semi-skimmed (low-fat)	250 ml (8 fl oz)	12	12	4	Very Limited

Food	Portion	Total Carbs (g)	Total Sugar (g)	Total Fat (g)	Recmmd.
Longlife/UHT whole milk	250 ml (8 fl oz)	12	12	10	Avoid
Goat's milk	250 ml (8 fl oz)	11	11	9	Avoid
Canned milk					
Evaporated, low-fat	2 tbsp	3	3	1	Good
Evaporated, whole	2 tbsp	2.5	2.5	2.5	Avoid
Sweetened condensed skimmed	2 tbsp	19	19	Tr	Avoid
Sweetened condensed, regular	2 tbsp	17	17	3	Avoid
Dried milk					
Skimmed	30 g (1 oz)	16	16	Tr	Good
Whole	30 g (1 oz)	13	13	8	Avoid
Soya milk					
Flavoured	250 ml (8 fl oz)	26	23	6	Avoid
Natural, unsweetened	250 ml (8 fl oz)	1	0.5	4	Good
Natural, sweetened	250 ml (8 fl oz)	6	5	6	Limited
Rice drink	250 ml (8 fl oz)	24	13	3	Very Limited
Oat/cereal drink	250 ml (8 fl oz)	16	10	4	Limited

MILK, MILK PRODUCTS AND MILK SUBSTITUTES (CONT.)
YOGURTS

Food	Portion	Total Carbs (g)	Total Sugar (g)	Total Fat (g)	Recmmd.
Fruit					
Fat-free, sweetened	125 g (4½ oz)	9	8	Tr	Avoid
Low-fat, sweetened	125 g (4½ oz)	17	16	1	Avoid
Whole milk, sweetened	125 g (4½ oz)	22	21	4	Avoid
Bio yogurt	125 g (4½ oz)	22	21	4	Avoid
Natural					
Fat-free	125 g (4½ oz)	8	8	Tr	Good
Low-fat	125 g (4½ oz)	8	8	1	Limited
Whole milk	125 g (4½ oz)	10	10	4	Avoid
Bio yogurt, whole milk	125 g (4½ oz)	10	10	3	Avoid
Drinks					
Fat-free, probiotic	200 ml (7 fl oz)	14	10	Tr	Limited
Whole milk, sweetened	200 ml (7 fl oz)	28	28	3	Avoid
Fermented milk drink (e.g.Yakult)	65 ml (2¼ fl oz)	18	18	Tr	Limited
Soya yogurt	125 g (4½ oz)	5	4	5	Good

NUTS, NUT BUTTERS AND SEEDS

News of the positive health benefits of nuts continues to accumulate. Nuts are a great source of good fats and protein, and consumption of nuts has been associated with decreased risks of heart attacks. Almonds, Brazil nuts, peanuts, pistachios, and many other nuts are all good choices. Natural nut butters appear to have the same health benefits as whole nuts, but it is important to read the labels to make sure that hydrogenated oils are not listed as ingredients.

NUTS, SHELLED

Food	Portion	Total Carbs (g)	Total Sugar (g)	Total Fat (g)	Recmmd.
Almonds	30 g (1 oz)	2	1	17	Good
Brazil nuts	30 g (1 oz)	1	0.5	20	Good
Cashews, roasted	30 g (1 oz)	6	2	15	Good
Chestnuts, roasted	30 g (1 oz)	11	2	1	Limited
Chestnuts, canned or vacuum-packed	30 g (1 oz)	11	2	1	Limited
Coconut, fresh flesh	30 g (1 oz)	1	1	10	Limited
Coconut, desiccated, unsweetened	30 g (1 oz)	2	2	19	Very Limited
Hazelnuts	30 g (1 oz)	2	1	19	Good
Macadamias	30 g (1 oz)	1.5	1	23	Good
Peanuts, roasted	30 g (1 oz)	2	1	16	Good
Pecans	30 g (1 oz)	2	1	21	Good
Pine nuts	30 g (1 oz)	1	1	20	Good
Pistachios	30 g (1 oz)	2	1.5	17	Good
Walnuts	30 g (1 oz)	1	1	20	Good

NUT BUTTERS AND PURÉES

Food	Portion	Total Carbs (g)	Total Sugar (g)	Total Fat (g)	Recmmd.
Almond butter	1 tbsp	3	1	10	Good
Cashew butter	1 tbsp	4	1	9	Good
Chestnut purée	30 g (1 oz)	7	Tr	Tr	Limited
Chestnut purée sweetened	30 g (1 oz)	8	2	Tr	Very Limited
Coconut cream, block	30 g (1 oz)	2	2	21	Avoid
Coconut milk, unsweetened	2 tbsp	1.5	0.5	5	Limited
Hazelnut butter	1 tbsp	3	1	11	Good
Peanut butter, reduced-fat	1 tbsp	6	2	7	Good
Peanut butter, no added sugar	1 tbsp	2	1	10	Good
Tahini (sesame seed paste)	1 tbsp	Tr	Tr	12	Good

SEEDS

Food	Portion	Total Carbs (g)	Total Sugar (g)	Total Fat (g)	Recmmd.
Linseed (flaxseed)	1 tbsp	3	Tr	5	Good
Poppy	1 tbsp	3	Tr	6	Good
Pumpkin	1 tbsp	2	Tr	7	Good
Sesame	1 tbsp	Tr	Tr	9	Good
Sunflower	1 tbsp	3	Tr	7	Good

PASTA AND PASTA DISHES

Wholewheat pasta is the preferred type of pasta on the South Beach Diet. We recommend that you boil the pasta until just tender or 'al dente'. Also, to reduce portion size, try eating pasta as a side dish to your fish or chicken, rather than a meal in itself.

Enjoy your pasta with a low-sugar tomato sauce. Research shows that lycopene in tomatoes can be more efficiently absorbed when processed into tomato sauces or tomato paste. This is important because lycopene has been shown to help prevent prostate cancer.

PASTA, COOKED – 90 g dried pasta gives 230 g cooked

Food	Portion	Total Carbs (g)	Total Sugar (g)	Total Fat (g)	Recmmd.
Capelli d'angelo durum wheat	230 g (8 oz)	45	1	1	Very Limited
Corn pasta	230 g (8 oz)	45	2	2	Avoid
Egg noodles, fresh, plain, spinach, or tomato	230 g (8 oz)	30	0.5	1	Very Limited
Fettuccine, egg noodle, spinach	230 g (8 oz)	30	0.5	1	Very Limited
Pasta shells and spirals	230 g (8 oz)	45	1	1	Very Limited
Linguine, durum wheat	230 g (8 oz)	45	1	1	Very Limited
Macaroni, durum wheat	230 g (8 oz)	45	1	1	Very Limited
Macaroni, wholewheat	230 g (8 oz)	50	2	2	Very Limited
Spaghetti, durum wheat	230 g (8 oz)	51	1	2	Very Limited
Spaghetti, wholewheat	230 g (8 oz)	53	3	2	Limited

PASTA DISHES

Food	Portion	Total Carbs (g)	Total Sugar (g)	Total Fat (g)	Recmmd.
Gnocchi (potato dumplings)	200 g (7 oz)	35	2	0.5	Avoid
Filled pasta, without sauce					
ravioli, meat-filled	170 g (6 oz)	20	4	10	Avoid
tortellini, four-cheese	170 g (6 oz)	32	2	8	Avoid
tortellini, spinach and ricotta	170 g (6 oz)	32	2	7	Avoid
Lasagne, w/meat sauce, homemade	200 g (7 oz)	30	5	21	Very Limited
Lasagne, w/spinach, vegetarian, homemade	200 g (7 oz)	30	9	8	Very Limited
Macaroni cheese, canned	200 g (7 oz)	24	5	20	Avoid
Macaroni cheese, homemade	200 g (7 oz)	25	5	25	Avoid
Meat ravioli, w/meat sauce	200 g (7 oz)	25	5	15	Avoid
Meat ravioli, w/tomato sauce	200 g (7 oz)	20	4	4	Avoid
Spaghetti					
w/tomato sauce, canned	200 g (7 oz)	28	11	1	Very Limited

Food	Portion	Total Carbs (g)	Total Sugar (g)	Total Fat (g)	Recmmd.
w/tomato sauce, homemade	200 g (7 oz)	20	4	4	Limited
Bolognese	200 g (7 oz)	30	3	6	Avoid
Carbonara	200 g (7 oz)	25	22	24	Avoid
Tortellini, meat, w/chicken and mushroom sauce	200 g (7 oz)	35	3	6	Avoid
Tortellini, cheese, w/tomato sauce	200 g (7 oz)	35	3	7	Avoid

PICKLES, CHUTNEYS AND RELISHES

Pickles, peppers and relishes are all allowed on the South Beach Diet as long as they are not the sweetened versions.

Food	Portion	Total Carbs (g)	Total Sugar (g)	Total Fat (g)	Recmmd.
Apple/tomato chutney	1 tbsp	7	7	Tr	Limited
Branston pickle	1 tbsp	5	5	Tr	Limited
Chermoula	1 tbsp	0	0	9	Limited
Dill cucumber pickle	1 large, 90 g (3 oz)	2	2	Tr	Limited
Gherkin, sweet	1 medium, 40 g (1¼ oz)	1	1	Tr	Limited
Harissa paste	1 tbsp	0	0	8	Good
Jalapeño peppers, pickled	30 g (1 oz)	2	2	Tr	Limited
Lime pickle	1 tsp	Tr	Tr	Tr	Good

PICKLES, CHUTNEYS AND RELISHES (CONT.)

Food	Portion	Total Carbs (g)	Total Sugar (g)	Total Fat (g)	Recmmd.
Mango chutney	1 tbsp	7	7	2	Limited
Peppers, roasted, whole, red, in olive oil	30 g (1 oz)	8	7	2.5	Good
Piccalilli	1 tbsp	3	2	Tr	Limited
Pickled red cabbage	50 g (1¾ oz)	2	Tr	Tr	Good
Pickled walnuts	30 g (1 oz)	9	3	1	Good
Sauerkraut, drained	75 g (2½ oz)	1	1	Tr	Good
Sweetcorn relish	1 tbsp	4	4	Tr	Limited
Tomato chilli jam	1 tbsp	8	7	8	Limited

PIZZA

If pizza is among your favourite treats, choose thin-crust pizza with vegetable toppings: tomatoes, peppers, onions, mushrooms. Thick-crust pizzas, as well as those made on French bread, are trouble. Also steer clear of high saturated fat toppings, such as mixed cheeses, pepperoni and sausage. The tomato sauce found on most pizza may play a role in preventing prostate cancer thanks to lycopene, an antioxidant found in tomato products.

Food	Portion	Total Carbs (g)	Total Sugar (g)	Total Fat (g)	Recmmd.
Cheese and tomato French bread pizza	145 g (5 oz)	45	3	11	Avoid
Pizza base, 20 cm (8 in)	145 g (5 oz)	80	5	7	Avoid

PIZZA – All portions based on ¼ of a 30 cm (12 in) pizza

Food	Portion	Total Carbs (g)	Total Sugar (g)	Total Fat (g)	Recmmd.
Deep dish					
Cheese and tomato (margherita)	170 g (6 oz)	60	4	13	Avoid
Pepperoni	170 g (6 oz)	58	3	18	Avoid
Ham and pineapple	170 g (6 oz)	59	5	15	Avoid
Vegetable	170 g (6 oz)	58	4	12	Avoid
Thin crust					
Cheese and tomato (margherita)	125 g (4½ oz)	42	3	13	Limited
Four-cheese	150 g (5½ oz)	50	4	16	Avoid
Bacon and mushroom	150 g (5½ oz)	52	3	14	Avoid
Mixed meats	150 g (5½ oz)	43	3	16	Avoid
Chargrilled chicken	170 g (6 oz)	53	4	14	Avoid
Roasted vegetable	150 g (5½ oz)	44	3	10	Limited
Spinach and ricotta	150 g (5½ oz)	42	3	11	Limited
Seafood w/o cheese	150 g (5½ oz)	42	3	11	Limited

POULTRY AND GAME

When it comes to chicken, bake, grill, roast or sauté, but do not fry. Choose the breast meat, which has far less saturated fat than the leg, thigh and wing, and remove the skin before eating. For processed poultry products, see pages 93–4. Duck and goose are higher in saturated fat than chicken and should not be eaten often.

CHICKEN (AN AVERAGE OF LIGHT AND DARK MEAT)

Food	Portion	Total Carbs (g)	Total Sugar (g)	Total Fat (g)	Recmmd.
Fried, in batter	100 g (3½ oz)	18	1	20	Avoid
Fried, in breadcrumbs	100 g (3½ oz)	15	1	12	Avoid
Crispy crumbed, baked	100 g (3½ oz)	15	1	11	Avoid
Roasted, w/skin	100 g (3½ oz)	0	0	7	Very Limited
Roasted, without skin	100 g (3½ oz)	0	0	4	Good
Poached, w/skin	100 g (3½ oz)	0	0	5	Very Limited
Poached, without skin	100 g (3½ oz)	0	0	3	Good
Minced chicken	100 g (3½ oz)	0	0	3	Good

CHICKEN LIVERS

Food	Portion	Total Carbs (g)	Total Sugar (g)	Total Fat (g)	Recmmd.
Fried	100 g (3½ oz)	Tr	Tr	9	Avoid
Chicken liver paté	50 g (1¾ oz)	0.5	Tr	17	Avoid

CHICKEN PORTIONS

Food	Portion	Total Carbs (g)	Total Sugar (g)	Total Fat (g)	Recmmd.
Breast					
Fried, crumbed, w/skin	90 g (3 oz)	13	0.5	12	Avoid
Grilled	90 g (3 oz)	0	0	8	Good
Roasted, w/skin	1 breast, 90 g (3 oz)	0	0	5	Very Limited
Roasted, without skin	1 breast, 75 g (2½ oz)	0	0	2	Good
Tandoori, w/skin	100 g (3½ oz)	2	1	5	Very Limited
Drumstick					
Fried, crumbed, w/skin	75 g (2½ oz)	10	0.5	7	Avoid
Chinese-style	100 g (3½ oz)	4	4	10	Avoid
Roasted, w/skin	100 g (3½ oz)	0	0	9	Very Limited
Roasted, without skin	75 g (2½ oz)	0	0	3	Limited
BBQ, w/skin	75 g (2½ oz)	3	3	10	Very Limited
Thigh					
Roasted, w/skin	100 g (3½ oz)	0	0	16	Very Limited
Roasted, without skin	100 g (3½ oz)	0	0	9	Limited

POULTRY AND GAME (CONT.)

Food	Portion	Total Carbs (g)	Total Sugar (g)	Total Fat (g)	Recmmd.
Wings					
Chinese-style	100 g (3½ oz)	4	3	16	Avoid
Hot and spicy	100 g (3½ oz)	4	3	16	Avoid

CHICKEN DISHES

Food	Portion	Total Carbs (g)	Total Sugar (g)	Total Fat (g)	Recmmd.
Kiev, w/skin	150 g (5½ oz)	18	1	25	Avoid
W/black bean sauce	150 g (5½ oz)	15	6	8	Avoid
W/lemon sauce	150 g (5½ oz)	15	6	9	Avoid
W/red or white wine sauce	150 g (5½ oz)	4	1	14	Avoid
W/tomato and basil sauce	150 g (5½ oz)	3	1	6	Limited

TURKEY

Food	Portion	Total Carbs (g)	Total Sugar (g)	Total Fat (g)	Recmmd.
Dark meat, w/skin	100 g (3½ oz)	0	0	5	Very Limited
Dark meat, without skin	100 g (3½ oz)	0	0	3	Limited
Light meat, w/skin	100 g (3½ oz)	0	0	2	Limited
Light meat, without skin	100 g (3½ oz)	0	0	1	Good
Minced turkey breast	100 g (3½ oz)	0	0	1	Good

Food	Portion	Total Carbs (g)	Total Sugar (g)	Total Fat (g)	Recmmd.
Turkey, roasted					
Breast meat, w/skin	100 g (3½ oz)	0	0	2	Very Limited
Breast meat, without skin	100 g (3½ oz)	0	0	1	Good
Leg, w/skin	230 g (8 oz)	0	0	10	Very Limited
Leg, without skin	230 g (8 oz)	0	0	4	Limited

OTHER POULTRY

Food	Portion	Total Carbs (g)	Total Sugar (g)	Total Fat (g)	Recmmd.
Duck, roasted					
w/skin	100 g (3½ oz)	0	0	38	Very Limited
without skin	100 g (3½ oz)	0	0	10	Very Limited
Goose, roasted					
w/skin	100 g (3½ oz)	0	0	21	Very Limited
without skin	100 g (3½ oz)	0	0	15	Very Limited
Guinea fowl, roasted					
w/skin	100 g (3½ oz)	0	0	12	Very Limited
without skin	100 g (3½ oz)	0	0	8	Good
Quail	100 g (3½ oz)	0	0	5	Good

POULTRY AND GAME (CONT.)
GAME

Food	Portion	Total Carbs (g)	Total Sugar (g)	Total Fat (g)	Recmmd.
Grouse, roasted	100 g (3½ oz)	0	0	2	Good
Hare, roasted	100 g (3½ oz)	0	0	5	Good
Hare, jugged or stewed	100 g (3½ oz)	0	0	3	Good
Kangaroo	100 g (3½ oz)	1	1	2	Good
Ostrich	100 g (3½ oz)	0	0	3	Good
Pheasant, roasted	100 g (3½ oz)	0	0	3	Good
Pigeon, roasted	100 g (3½ oz)	0	0	8	Good
Pigeon breasts, without skin	100 g (3½ oz)	0	0	4	Good
Partridge, roasted	100 g (3½ oz)	0	0	4	Good
Rabbit, roasted	100 g (3½ oz)	0	0	5	Good
Rabbit, casserole	100 g (3½ oz)	0	0	3	Good
Venison haunch, roasted	100 g (3½ oz)	0	0	2	Good
Venison fillet medallions, grilled	100 g (3½ oz)	0	0	2	Good

SALADS AND SALAD DRESSINGS

Prepared salads, such as tuna or egg, can be an occasional part of your diet, but the best salads are those made with fresh salad leaves, crisp vegetables and a flavourful vinaigrette dressing.

SALADS

Food	Portion	Total Carbs (g)	Total Sugar (g)	Total Fat (g)	Recmmd.
Mixed bean salad	75 g (2½ oz)	10	2	7	Good
Caesar salad, w/dressing	100 g (3½ oz)	7	3	10	Good
Coleslaw, traditional, sweetened	50 g (1¾ oz)	2	2	13	Very Limited
Coleslaw, low-fat	50 g (1¾ oz)	3	3	2	Limited
Cucumber salad, marinated in vinaigrette dressing	50 g (1¾ oz)	Tr	Tr	5	Good
Egg mayonnaise	100 g (3½ oz)	1	1	20	Very Limited
Greek salad, w/olives and feta cheese	150 g (5½ oz)	3	1	19	Limited
Grilled chicken Caesar salad	150 g (5½ oz)	9	2	15	Good
Pasta salad, w/chargrilled vegetables	150 g (5½ oz)	20	2	10	Limited
Pasta salad w/prawns	150 g (5½ oz)	20	2	10	Limited
Potato salad	100 g (3½ oz)	11	1	26	Avoid
Tabbouleh	100 g (3½ oz)	17	2	5	Good

SALADS AND SALAD DRESSINGS (CONT.)

Food	Portion	Total Carbs (g)	Total Sugar (g)	Total Fat (g)	Recmmd.
Tomato salad, w/mozzarella	100 g (3½ oz)	2	2	18	Good
Tomato and avocado salad	150 g (5½ oz)	3	2	18	Good
Tossed green salad, w/carrot, cucumber and tomato	30 g (1 oz)	Tr	Tr	2	Good
Tuna niçoise salad	150 g (5½ oz)	9	6	13	Good
Waldorf salad	100 g (3½ oz)	8	1	17	Avoid

SALAD DRESSINGS

Food	Portion	Total Carbs (g)	Total Sugar (g)	Total Fat (g)	Recmmd.
Blue cheese, reduced-fat	1 tbsp	2	2	4	Good
Blue cheese, regular	1 tbsp	1.5	1.5	7	Limited
Caesar-style, reduced-fat	1 tbsp	2	2	4	Good
Caesar, regular	1 tbsp	2	2	6	Good

Food	Portion	Total Carbs (g)	Total Sugar (g)	Total Fat (g)	Recmmd.
French					
Reduced-fat	1 tbsp	1.5	1.5	Tr	Limited
Regular	1 tbsp	1	1	7	Avoid
Italian					
Reduced-fat	1 tbsp	1.5	1.5	Tr	Good
Regular	1 tbsp	1	1	7	Good
Thousand Island					
Fat-free	1 tbsp	2	2	Tr	Limited
Regular	1 tbsp	2	2	5	Very Limited
Vinaigrette, balsamic, regular	1 tbsp	1	1	7	Good
Vinaigrette, olive oil and wine vinegar, homemade	1 tbsp	1	1	7	Good
Mayonnaise					
Light	1 tbsp	2	1	3	Limited
Reduced-calorie	1 tbsp	2	1	4	Limited
Regular	1 tbsp	0.5	Tr	11	Limited
Salad cream					
Light	1 tbsp	1	1	3	Limited
Regular	1 tbsp	2.5	2.5	5	Very Limited

SAUCES, GRAVIES AND STOCKS

Canned and ready-made gravies and sauces are often very high in fat and salt, and some sauces contain added sweeteners such as sugar, honey or syrup, so read the list of ingredients carefully before you buy.

When serving meat or poultry, make gravy with the cooking juices, skimming off the fat, then heightening the flavour with a squeeze of lemon or lime juice, a touch of mustard or a dash of hot-pepper sauce.

CONDIMENTS

Food	Portion	Total Carbs (g)	Total Sugar (g)	Total Fat (g)	Recmmd.
Brown sauce	1 tbsp	3	3	Tr	Avoid
Chilli sauce, sweetened	1 tbsp	6	5	Tr	Avoid
Chilli and garlic sauce, unsweetened	1 tbsp	2	2	Tr	Limited
Cranberry sauce	1 tbsp	10	10	0	Avoid
Cumberland sauce	1 tbsp	10	9	Tr	Avoid
Dill (gravadlax) sauce	1 tbsp	4	4	2	Avoid
Horseradish	2 tsp	3	2	1	Good
Horseradish, creamed	2 tsp	3	2	2	Limited
Hot-pepper sauce	1 tsp	Tr	Tr	Tr	Good
Lemon juice	1 tbsp	Tr	Tr	Tr	Good
Lime juice	1 tbsp	Tr	Tr	Tr	Good
Mint sauce	1 tsp	1.5	1.5	Tr	Good
Mustard, made	1 tsp	0.5	0.5	0.5	Good
Redcurrant jelly	1 tbsp	10	9	0	Avoid
Soy sauce	1 tsp	0.5	0.5	Tr	Limited

Food	Portion	Total Carbs (g)	Total Sugar (g)	Total Fat (g)	Recmmd.
Tartare sauce	1 tbsp	3	2.5	4	Avoid
Tomato ketchup, sweetened	1 tbsp	4	4	Tr	Avoid
Vinegar	1 tbsp	Tr	Tr	0	Good
Worcestershire sauce	1 tsp	1	1	Tr	Good

GRAVIES, STOCKS AND PASTES

Food	Portion	Total Carbs (g)	Total Sugar (g)	Total Fat (g)	Recmmd.
Beef stock cube	1 cube, 10 g	1	Tr	1	Limited
Beef stock, fresh	4 tbsp	1	Tr	1	Good
Bovril	1 tsp	Tr	Tr	Tr	Good
Chicken stock, fresh	4 tbsp	1	Tr	1.5	Good
Chicken stock cube	1 cube, 10 g	1	Tr	1.5	Limited
Fish stock, fresh	4 tbsp	1	Tr	1	Good
Fish stock cube	1 cube, 10 g	1	Tr	1	Limited
Homemade gravy, thickened with flour	4 tbsp	5	1	6	Very Limited
Gravy granules, prepared w/water	4 tbsp	2	Tr	1.5	Very Limited
Vegetable bouillon powder	1 tbsp	1	Tr	1	Limited
Vegetable stock cube	1 cube, 10 g	1	Tr	2	Limited

SAUCES, GRAVIES AND STOCKS (CONT.)

Food	Portion	Total Carbs (g)	Total Sugar (g)	Total Fat (g)	Recmmd.
Yeast extract (e.g. Marmite, Vegemite)	1 tsp	Tr	Tr	Tr	Good

SAUCES

Food	Portion	Total Carbs (g)	Total Sugar (g)	Total Fat (g)	Recmmd.
Apple sauce					
unsweetened	2 tbsp	3	3	Tr	Limited
w/sugar	2 tbsp	8	7	Tr	Avoid
Barbecue sauce	4 tbsp	14	14	Tr	Avoid
Béarnaise	4 tbsp	7	5	20	Avoid
Béchamel (white sauce)					
thin, made with skimmed milk	4 tbsp	5	2	3	Limited
thin, made with semi-skimmed (low-fat) milk	4 tbsp	5	2	4	Very Limited
thick, made with semi-skimmed (low-fat) milk	4 tbsp	9	4	6	Avoid
thick, made with whole milk	4 tbsp	9	4	8	Avoid
Bolognese	170 g (6 oz)	4	4	20	Avoid
Bread sauce					
made with semi-skimmed (low-fat) milk	3 tbsp	7	2	1	Avoid

Food	Portion	Total Carbs (g)	Total Sugar (g)	Total Fat (g)	Recmmd.
made with whole milk	3 tbsp	7	2	2	Avoid
Carbonara	150 g (5½ oz)	5	0.5	18	Avoid
Cheese sauce					
made with semi-skimmed (low-fat) milk	4 tbsp	5	2	8	Very Limited
made with whole milk	4 tbsp	5	2	9	Avoid
Cheese fondue, homemade	4 tbsp	12	6	20	Avoid
Cook-in sauce					
curry	150 g (5½ oz)	11	6	7	Avoid
sweet and sour	150 g (5½ oz)	15	8	1	Avoid
white wine	150 g (5½ oz)	12	7	2	Avoid
Hoisin sauce	1 tbsp	7	7	Tr	Avoid
Hollandaise sauce	4 tbsp	0	0	40	Avoid
Onion sauce					
made with semi-skimmed (low-fat) milk	4 tbsp	5	2	3	Very Limited
made with whole milk	4 tbsp	5	2	4	Avoid
Oyster sauce	1 tbsp	3	2	0	Limited
Parsley sauce					
made with semi-skimmed (low-fat) milk	4 tbsp	5	2	3	Very Limited

SAUCES (CONT.)

Food	Portion	Total Carbs (g)	Total Sugar (g)	Total Fat (g)	Recmmd.
made with whole milk	4 tbsp	5	2	4	Avoid
Red wine sauce	4 tbsp	6	4	Tr	Very Limited
Salsa, homemade	2 tbsp	2	2	0.5	Good
Salsa, from a jar	4 tbsp	4	3	1	Good
Satay (peanut) sauce	2 tbsp	6	4	6	Good
Seafood sauce	1 tbsp	2	2	6	Avoid
Stir-fry sauce					
balti	3 tbsp	3	2	2	Avoid
black bean	3 tbsp	9	7	0.5	Avoid
lemon	3 tbsp	10	10	0.5	Avoid
sweet and sour	3 tbsp	10	10	1.5	Avoid
Sweet and sour	150 g (5½ oz)	15	8	1	Avoid
Teriyaki sauce	2 tbsp	6	6	Tr	Very Limited
Tikka masala	150 g (5½ oz)	15	12	12	Avoid
Tomato-based pasta sauce, fresh	125 g (4½ oz)	5	4	2.5	Limited
Tomato-based pasta sauce, from a jar	125 g (4½ oz)	9	7	5	Limited
Tomato passata (sieved tomatoes)	125 g (4½ oz)	8	7	Tr	Good

SOUPS

A first course of soup will not only soothe your spirits, it will satisfy your appetite. Research shows that people given a first course of tomato soup ate less during subsequent courses. Good choices also include vegetable soups, such as bean, gazpacho or lentil, which are all packed with good carbs and fibre.

Avoid cream-type soups in restaurants because they are usually made with saturated fat-laden cream or whole milk. At home, make cream-type soups with water. When ordering French onion soup you might want to order it without the French bread and cheese topping.

Food	Portion	Total Carbs (g)	Total Sugar (g)	Total Fat (g)	Recmmd.
Beef and vegetable	250 ml (8 fl oz)	17	3	2	Good
Beef consommé	250 ml (8 fl oz)	2	1	Tr	Good
Black bean	250 ml (8 fl oz)	17	7	5	Good
Bouillabaisse	250 ml (8 fl oz)	10	2	5	Good
Broccoli and Stilton	250 ml (8 fl oz)	9	3	9	Very Limited
Carrot and coriander	250 ml (8 fl oz)	15	6	6	Good
Chicken noodle	250 ml (8 fl oz)	7	1	1	Very Limited
Chicken and sweetcorn	250 ml (8 fl oz)	10	3	10	Very Limited
Cream of asparagus	250 ml (8 fl oz)	15	4	11	Avoid
Cream of chicken	250 ml (8 fl oz)	11	3	10	Avoid
Cream of mushroom	250 ml (8 fl oz)	10	2	8	Avoid

SOUPS (CONT.)

Food	Portion	Total Carbs (g)	Total Sugar (g)	Total Fat (g)	Recmmd.
Cream of tomato	250 ml (8 fl oz)	15	7	8	Limited
French onion soup	250 ml (8 fl oz)	11	7	2	Limited
Gazpacho	250 ml (8 fl oz)	15	7	2	Good
Lentil	250 ml (8 fl oz)	25	4	5	Good
Lentil and bacon	250 ml (8 fl oz)	20	3	3	Good
Lobster bisque	250 ml (8 fl oz)	9	4	5	Avoid
Minestrone	250 ml (8 fl oz)	15	3	2	Good
Miso broth	250 ml (8 fl oz)	2	1	Tr	Good
Pea and mint	250 ml (8 fl oz)	20	2	3	Limited
Scotch broth	250 ml (8 fl oz)	20	2	3	Good
Spicy parsnip	250 ml (8 fl oz)	12	4	1	Limited
Tomato	250 ml (8 fl oz)	15	7	2	Good
Vegetable	250 ml (8 fl oz)	22	10	2	Good
Vichyssoise	250 ml (8 fl oz)	16	5	7	Limited

SUGARS, JAMS AND SWEETENERS

Naturally occurring sugars are those found in foods like milk products (lactose) and fruits (fructose). Refined sugars include honey, maple syrup, and table sugar. Most sugars have a low to moderate ranking on the glycaemic index. Table sugar (sucrose) has a moderate ranking and can be included as part of an occasional treat or as an ingredient in baking.

However, sugar is the number one additive to our food supply. The typical person eats approximately 32 teaspoons of added sugar a day. Some glucose syrup may be added even to products using sugar substitutes. Read and compare labels and choose wisely.

CANE SUGAR

Food	Portion	Total Carbs (g)	Total Sugar (g)	Total Fat (g)	Recmmd.
Demerara sugar	1 tbsp	20	20	0	Very Limited
Muscovado sugar	1 tbsp	20	20	0	Very Limited
White sugar	1 tsp	5	5	0	Very Limited
	1 tbsp	15	15	0	Avoid
	100 g (3½ oz)	100	100	0	Avoid

JAMS, JELLIES AND FRUIT SPREADS

Food	Portion	Total Carbs (g)	Total Sugar (g)	Total Fat (g)	Recmmd.
Fig preserve	1 tbsp	10	10	0	Avoid
Fruit conserve (high-fruit jam)	1 tbsp	10	10	0	Avoid
Jam or jelly					
reduced sugar	1 tbsp	5	5	0	Very Limited
regular	1 tbsp	10	10	0	Avoid
sugar-free	1 tbsp	5	0	0	Avoid
Lemon curd	1 tbsp	9	6	1	Avoid
Marmalade, orange					
reduced sugar	1 tbsp	5	5	0	Very Limited
regular	1 tbsp	10	10	0	Avoid
Melon preserve	1 tbsp	10	10	0	Avoid
Pure fruit spread	1 tbsp	5	5	0	Very Limited

SUGARS, JAMS AND SWEETENERS (CONT.)
OTHER SUGARS

Food	Portion	Total Carbs (g)	Total Sugar (g)	Total Fat (g)	Recmmd.
Fruit sugar (fructose)	2 tsp	10	10	0	Good
Glucose	2 tsp	10	10	0	Avoid

SUGAR SUBSTITUTES

Food	Portion	Total Carbs (g)	Total Sugar (g)	Total Fat (g)	Recmmd.
Aspartame (e.g. Canderel Spoonful, Equal)	1 tsp	0.5	0	0	Allowed
Sucralose (e.g. Splenda)	1 tsp	0.5	0	0	Allowed

SYRUPS

Food	Portion	Total Carbs (g)	Total Sugar (g)	Total Fat (g)	Recmmd.
Black treacle	1 tbsp	10	10	0	Avoid
Glucose syrup	1 tbsp	13	13	0	Avoid
Golden syrup	1 tbsp	12	12	0	Avoid
Honey	1 tbsp	11	11	0	Very Limited
Maple syrup, pure	1 tbsp	12	12	0	Very Limited
Maple-flavoured syrup	1 tbsp	12	12	0	Avoid
Pancake syrup, reduced-calorie	1 tbsp	6	6	0	Avoid

VEGETABLES AND HERBS

Eat and enjoy plenty of vegetables. They are low in calories but high in vitamins, minerals and other essential nutrients, plus fibre. Brightly coloured green, red and yellow vegetables contain antioxidants, such as vitamins A, C and E. Opt for as much variety as possible: carrots are fine, but sweetcorn should be limited, because of its high carbohydrate content. In addition to their nutrient contribution, vegetables, especially when eaten raw, are a great source of fibre and bulk. When cooked in water, vegetables quickly lose their nutrients: use as little water as possible, and cook for as short a time as possible. For canned and dried beans and pulses, see page 31.

Food	Portion	Total Carbs (g)	Total Sugar (g)	Total Fat (g)	Recmmd.
Alfalfa sprouts, raw	50 g (1¾ oz)	2	1	Tr	Good
Artichokes, Chinese, cooked	100 g (3½ oz)	17	10	Tr	Limited
Artichokes, globe, edible portion	50 g (1¾ oz)	1	0	0	Good
Artichokes, Jerusalem, cooked	100 g (3½ oz)	12	8	Tr	Good
Asparagus, cooked	5 spears, 125 g (4½ oz)	2	2	1	Good
Aubergine (eggplant), cooked	½ medium, 125 g (4½ oz)	3	3	0.5	Good
Avocado	½, 75 g (2½ oz)	1.5	0.5	15	Good
Basil	2 tbsp	Tr	Tr	Tr	Good
Beans, broad	100 g (3½ oz)	12	1.5	0.5	Limited
Beans, green	75 g (2½ oz)	4	2	Tr	Good

VEGETABLES AND HERBS (CONT.)

Food	Portion	Total Carbs (g)	Total Sugar (g)	Total Fat (g)	Recmmd.
Bean sprouts, mung, raw	40 g (1¼ oz)	2	1	Tr	Good
Beetroot, raw	75 g (2½ oz)	6	5	Tr	Very Limited
Beetroot, boiled	75 g (2½ oz)	7	6	Tr	Very Limited
Beetroot, pickled	75 g (2½ oz)	4	4	Tr	Limited
Broccoli, boiled	90 g (3 oz)	1	1	1	Good
Brussels sprouts, boiled	10 sprouts, 100 g (3½ oz)	3	3	1	Good
Butternut squash, cooked	100 g (3½ oz)	8	7	Tr	Very Limited
Cabbage, green or red, boiled	100 g (3½ oz)	2	2	0.5	Good
Cabbage, white, raw	50 g (1¾ oz)	2.5	2.5	Tr	Good
Carrots, raw	4 small, 100 g (3½ oz)	8	7	Tr	Good
Carrots, boiled	4 small, 100 g (3½ oz)	5	4.5	Tr	Good
Cauliflower, raw	100 g (3½ oz)	3	2.5	1	Good
Cauliflower, cooked	100 g (3½ oz)	2	2	1	Good
Celeriac, raw	100 g (3½ oz)	4	3	Tr	Good
Celery, raw	1 stick, 30 g (1 oz)	Tr	Tr	Tr	Good
Chicory, raw	1 head, 30 g (1 oz)	Tr	Tr	Tr	Good

Food	Portion	Total Carbs (g)	Total Sugar (g)	Total Fat (g)	Recmmd.
Chilli, fresh, chopped	1 tbsp	Tr	Tr	Tr	Good
Chinese leaf, raw	100 g (3½ oz)	2	2	Tr	Good
Chives, chopped	2 tbsp	Tr	Tr	Tr	Good
Coriander, chopped	2 tbsp	Tr	Tr	Tr	Good
Courgettes (zucchini), raw	100 g (3½ oz)	2	2	0.5	Good
Cucumber, raw	30 g (1 oz)	0.5	0.5	0	Good
Endive, raw	30 g (1 oz)	1	0	0	Good
Fennel, raw	½ bulb, 115 g (4 oz)	2	2	Tr	Good
Garlic	1 clove	1	Tr	Tr	Good
Ginger, grated	1 tsp	Tr	Tr	Tr	Good
Jicama, raw	100 g (3½ oz)	8	1.5	Tr	Good
Kale, boiled	100 g (3½ oz)	1	1	1	Good
Kohlrabi	100 g (3½ oz)	3	2	Tr	Good
Leeks, trimmed and boiled	100 g (3½ oz)	2.5	2	0.5	Good
Lettuce, raw	30 g (1 oz)	0.5	0.5	Tr	Good
Mushrooms, raw	50 g (1¾ oz)	Tr	Tr	Tr	Good
Mustard cress	30 g (1 oz)	Tr	Tr	Tr	Good
Okra	8–10 pods, 90 g (3 oz)	2.5	2.5	1	Good
Onions, white or red, raw	100 g (3½ oz)	8	6	Tr	Good
Pak choi (bok choy), raw	100 g (3½ oz)	1	1	1	Good

VEGETABLES AND HERBS (CONT.)

Food	Portion	Total Carbs (g)	Total Sugar (g)	Total Fat (g)	Recmmd.
Parsley	2 tbsp	1	Tr	0.5	Good
Parsnips, cooked	100 g (3½ oz)	13	6	1	Very Limited
Peas					
Green, fresh or frozen, cooked	75 g (2½ oz)	8	1	1	Limited
Mangetouts (snow peas), cooked	75 g (2½ oz)	2.5	2	Tr	Good
Sugar snap, cooked	75 g (2½ oz)	2.5	2	Tr	Good
Pepper (capsicum), red, green, yellow or orange, raw	75 g (2½ oz)	4	4	Tr	Good
Potatoes, baked, w/skin					
Large	250 g (9 oz)	45	2	Tr	Avoid
Medium	150 g (5½ oz)	27	1	Tr	Avoid
Potatoes, other					
Instant mashed	60 g (2 oz)	8	0.5	Tr	Avoid
Mashed, regular, plain, no fat	60 g (2 oz)	9	0.5	Tr	Avoid
New, whole, boiled	75 g (2½ oz)	11	1	Tr	Very Limited
Potato gnocchi	100 g (3½ oz)	17	1	Tr	Avoid
Potatoes, roast	75 g (2½ oz)	19	0.5	3	Avoid
Potato skins	75 g (2½ oz)	22	Tr	Tr	Avoid

Food	Portion	Total Carbs (g)	Total Sugar (g)	Total Fat (g)	Recmmd.
Pumpkin and winter squash	100 g (3½ oz)	2	1.5	Tr	Avoid
Purple sprouting broccoli, boiled	90 g (3 oz)	1	1	1	Good
Radicchio, raw	30 g (1 oz)	1	1	Tr	Good
Radish, red	5, 40 g (1¼ oz)	1	1	Tr	Good
Radish, white (mooli, daikon)	50 g (1¾ oz)	1	1	Tr	Good
Ratatouille	200 g (7 oz)	7	7	10	Limited
Rocket	100 g (3½ oz)	1	1	0	Good
Sauerkraut	1 tbsp	Tr	Tr	Tr	Good
Shallots, chopped	2 tbsp	3	2	Tr	Good
Sorrel	30 g (1 oz)	Tr	Tr	Tr	Good
Spinach, cooked	100 g (3½ oz)	1	1	1	Good
Spinach, raw	30 g (1 oz)	Tr	Tr	Tr	Good
Spring or salad onions	3, 30 g (1 oz)	1	1	Tr	Good
Squash, yellow summer	100 g (3½ oz)	2	2	Tr	Good
Swede, cooked	60 g (2 oz)	2	2	Tr	Very Limited
Sweet potato, baked	60 g (2 oz)	12	7	Tr	Good
Sweetcorn, boiled	1 cob, 125 g (4½ oz)	25	3	3	Very Limited
Swiss chard	100 g (3½ oz)	3	3	Tr	Good
Tomato, ripe, raw	90 g (3 oz)	3	3	Tr	Good

VEGETABLES AND HERBS (CONT.)

Food	Portion	Total Carbs (g)	Total Sugar (g)	Total Fat (g)	Recmmd.
Tomatoes, canned, chopped	200 g (7 oz)	6	5	Tr	Good
Tomato juice, unsweetened	250 ml (8 fl oz)	8	8	Tr	Good
Tomato passata (sieved tomatoes)	200 g (7 oz)	12	10	Tr	Good
Tomato purée (concentrate)	2 tbsp	4	4	Tr	Good
Tomatoes, sun-dried	30 g (1 oz)	4	2	0	Good
Tomatoes, sun-dried, in oil	30 g (1 oz)	4	2	5	Good
Turnips, cooked	100 g (3½ oz)	2	2	Tr	Good
Water chestnuts, canned, drained	30 g (1 oz)	3	0.5	Tr	Good
Watercress	30 g (1 oz)	Tr	Tr	Tr	Good

THE SOUTH BEACH SUPERMARKET CHEAT SHEET

There's nothing worse than arriving home from work hungry and discovering that the cupboard is bare. Keep the following staple items in stock, and you'll always have the makings of a healthy South Beach meal.

Dairy Foods

Reduced-fat cheese An increasingly wide variety of cheeses is available in light, low-fat and reduced-fat versions. Experiment with different brands until you find the ones you like best.

Fat-free natural yogurt Use it for making creamy sauces (but don't let it boil) or dips (to thicken it, put it in a sieve lined with cheesecloth or a coffee filter and refrigerate it for 3 or more hours, then add your favourite herbs or seasonings).

Flavour Boosters

Balsamic vinegar It wakes up salad dressings, adds a rich flavour to sautés, and is great combined with olive oil in marinades.

Garlic No well-stocked kitchen is complete without garlic, a staple of Mediterranean cuisine.

Olive and rapeseed (canola) oils For the best-tasting salad dressings, light sautéing, dips for bread or crudités, or dressing for steamed vegetables, buy extra virgin olive oil. Rapeseed (canola) oil is good for stir-fries.

Onions Keep a couple of these in your vegetable rack: red, yellow or white onions; shallots; spring onions.

Salsa Use fresh or jarred salsa in place of ketchup and as an accompaniment for grilled meat, poultry or seafood.

Sesame oil and light soy sauce These add instant Asian flavour to steamed vegetables, stir-fries and marinades. Choose reduced-sodium soy sauce if available. Keep them in the refrigerator to help preserve their flavour if you don't use them up quickly.

Meat, Poultry and Fish

Sirloin steak For quick beef-and-vegetable kebabs, skewer the meat with mushrooms and chunks of red pepper and onion.

Boneless turkey and chicken breast Remove the skin, then grill, barbecue or bake the meat, or use it in stir-fries.

Prawns Stir-fry with vegetables, or add to a tomato and garlic sauce.

Salmon steaks Grill, poach, or wrap in foil with herbs and bake.

Vegetables and Pulses

Pulses Tinned beans, chickpeas and lentils are ready to use. Dried lentils and split peas are quick to cook as they don't need to be soaked overnight.

Frozen vegetables Keep broccoli and cauliflower florets, asparagus, green beans and spinach in the freezer for stir-fries, sautéed or microwaved side dishes, additions to casseroles and soups and dishes such as ratatouille.

Prewashed, prepackaged broccoli florets Serve them as no-fuss crudités with low-fat cheese or a yogurt dip, sauté them with black beans as a side dish, or add them to a ready-made soup.

Tinned tomatoes Don't be without them.

MENU MAKEOVERS

It's one thing to follow a straight-from-the-book diet plan, quite another to assemble your own healthy meals. But it's not as hard as it may seem. Simply pair a serving of lean protein with a serving of fibre-rich fresh vegetables (other than high-glycaemic varieties like sweetcorn and potatoes). Add a dash of healthy oils. Hey presto – you've got a delicious meal that slows your digestion and keeps you feeling satisfied for hours.

These before-and-after breakfast, lunch and dinner 'makeovers' will inspire you to think of your own tempting combinations.

SWITCH FROM THIS . . .	. . . TO THIS
BREAKFAST	
Fried egg, mushrooms, sautéed potatoes, bacon or pork sausage, and orange juice	Vegetable omelette, lean bacon, an orange, and skimmed milk
Croissant and a latte	One slice wholemeal toast with unsweetened peanut butter and coffee with skimmed milk
Cornflakes with whole milk and sugar	High-fibre bran cereal with skimmed milk and fresh fruit
LUNCH	
Salad with fat-free dressing and lasagne	Salad with olive oil and vinegar dressing (vinaigrette) and whole-wheat pasta with prawns and vegetables
Cheeseburger and fries	Grilled chicken breast sandwich on a multigrain roll
Roasted vegetable wrap	Avocado and bean salad wrapped in lettuce
DINNER	
Fried chicken, white rice and sweetcorn	Baked chicken breast, steamed asparagus and a tossed salad with vinaigrette
Meat pie and mashed potatoes	Grilled sirloin steak, sweet potato and oven-roasted vegetables
Cheese and pepperoni pizza, and a tossed salad with fat-free dressing	Tomato soup, open-faced roast beef sandwich and a tossed salad with vinaigrette

THE SOUTH BEACH DINING-OUT GUIDE

You don't have to stop frequenting your favourite restaurants just because you're on the South Beach Diet. This way of eating is flexible so that you can find several healthy choices that allow you to enjoy the dining-out experience and still lose or maintain weight. The following guidelines will help you select the healthiest choices virtually anywhere.

Regardless of which Phase of the Diet you're on, be guided by the ground rules for South Beach eating.

Chain Restaurants, Bars and Pubs

Chargrilled tuna, chicken or roasted vegetables are good healthy choices. Spinach and avocado salad with a small amount of grilled lean bacon or chicken makes a great starter or main course.

The salad bar contains all the ingredients for a healthy meal: fresh lettuce and spinach, chickpeas and bean salads, crisp fresh vegetables such as cauliflower, diced turkey or ham, olive oil and balsamic dressing.

Garlic mushrooms, unfortunately, are more likely to be cooked in butter or another unhealthy fat than in olive oil. Avoid deep-fried starters, as well as those that come smothered in cheese and sour cream (such as nachos or potato skins), sandwiches called melts (which are loaded with cheese), filled croissants, coleslaw, pasta and potato salads.

Chinese Food

Start with a hot and sour soup or a clear crab or chicken soup, and follow with steamed fish with ginger and spring onions or any combination of steamed vegetables prepared with small amounts of meat, poultry or seafood. Stir-fried dishes *should* be healthy, but often are not – request that a minimum of fat is used.

Stay away from: steamed rice (it has a high glycaemic index); deep-fried crispy noodles; spring rolls; fried dumplings; spareribs; chow mein; Peking duck; and dishes described on the menu as 'crispy' or 'sweet and sour'. Ask that your food be prepared without monosodium glutamate (MSG), the flavouring agent often used in Chinese restaurants, as it has a very high glycaemic index. Also, ask the waiter which sauces are prepared without cornflour.

Greek Food

Classic Mediterranean cooking is based on healthy olive oil, fresh vegetables, fish and meat, so there are plenty of choices for South Beach dieters. Fill up on Greek salad (lettuce, tomatoes, cucumbers, olives and feta cheese) and fish, meat (souvlakia) and vegetables cooked on a charcoal grill and enhanced with aromatic herbs and fresh lemon juice. Alternatively try stifado, a hearty meat stew with red wine, olive oil, onions and tomatoes.

Things to avoid are: dolmades (vine leaves stuffed with rice); calamari (squid) – because it's usually floured and deep-fried; and moussaka (vegetables layered with none-too-lean meat and covered with a thick, cheesy sauce).

Indian Food

Indian food is based on good carbs, particularly pulses like chickpeas and lentils, and vegetables such as spinach and aubergine (eggplant). The downside is its abundance of starchy carbs (breads, potatoes, rice, poppadums) and bad fats. Many appetizers are deep-fried, and vegetables and meats are typically fried or sautéed in the Indian butter called *ghee*. Still, most Indian restaurants provide several tasty choices for the South Beach dieter. Try mulligatawny soup; dals (lentil dishes – choose those without cream); chana (chickpea curry); kachumbars (vegetable salads); raitas (salads with a tart yogurt dressing); dishes described as dhansak (a combination of vegetables and lentils with herbs and spices) or tandoori (seasoned meat, poultry or fish roasted in a clay oven).

Stay away from samosas (deep-fried pastry filled with vegetables or meat); puri (a puffy, deep-fried bread) and dishes described as biryani, malai or korma, which are heavy on the oil and cream.

Italian Food

Not order pasta? At an Italian restaurant? Actually, it's easier than you think – there are usually several choices right for the South Beach dieter. Try the salads dressed with oil and balsamic vinegar; roasted peppers; clams or mussels steamed in white wine; clear soups; grilled meat, poultry, or fish; scallops sautéed with mushrooms and garlic; spinach or broccoli with garlic and olive oil.

If you order pizza, make sure you get thin-crust rather than deep-dish, cut right back on the cheese and pile it with vegetables rather than sausage or pepperoni. If you must have pasta, look for wholewheat pasta (*pasta integrale*). Order it as a side serving, with olive oil and garlic or topped with tomato sauce and good proteins (clams or prawns) or vegetables.

Stay away from bread and garlic bread; antipasti with cheeses and salami, which are high in saturated fat; anything with a rich cream and cheese sauce; and anything described as parmigiana (breadcrumbed or floured, fried and smothered in mozzarella and Parmesan).

Steak Houses

You should be able to have a good South Beach meal in a restaurant specializing in steaks and vegetables.

Try lean cuts of beef such as sirloin or fillet or a well-trimmed lamb or pork loin chop (ask that the extra fat be trimmed away before cooking). Ask for a side dish of steamed or grilled vegetables or a mixed salad dressed with olive oil and balsamic vinegar. As a first course, choose fresh shellfish, clear soup or a light salad.

Stay away from deep-fried appetizers, creamy soups, buttery and creamy sauces, coleslaw, pasta and potato salads, baked potatoes, fries and onion rings.

Thai Food

When you sit down in a Thai or Indonesian restaurant, you're often faced with the temptation of a plate of prawn crackers that are brought to your table: don't give in! They're made from a processed starch and deep-fried. Instead, order satay, little skewers of grilled chicken, pork, beef or tofu served with a peanut sauce. Good main course choices include steamed scallops or fish with a fragrant spicy sauce, or chicken stir-fried with basil. Traditional Thai green and red curries are often heavy on coconut milk, so they should be enjoyed in limited portions only. Avoid rice, rice noodles and egg noodles, but feel free to enjoy wun sen (cellophane or bean thread vermicelli), which have a low GI.

INDEX

Since the diet became popular in Miami and the book *The South Beach Diet* became a bestseller, I've heard from countless people eager to tell me about their weight loss successes. I'm encouraged by how easy the programme is to learn and put into practice. Now there is a website designed to make the diet even easier: *www.southbeachdiet.com.*

How? The website has the flexibility to provide personal feedback and guidance to help you reach your goals. It also has the ability to put you in touch with thousands of others following the plan. In the Message Boards, you'll be able to ask questions and get answers from a large community of dieters with similar experiences, as well as from our expert nutritionists. You'll get regular advice from me, too, in the Daily Dish newsletter and Ask Dr Agatston Q&As.

The site's interactive tools are also designed to provide personal support. In the WeightTracker, for instance, you can key in your weight, chart your progress, and get immediate feedback on how you're doing on the diet. The site will tell you if you're losing weight too fast or too slow, and what you can do about it. It's like having your own personal trainer pointing out areas for improvement, telling you that you're doing better than you think and keeping you motivated.

In the Meal Plans section of the site, you'll find Daily Menus for whatever phase of the diet you're in, a Recipe Search to help you find delicious new dishes quickly and easily (including vegetarian-only recipes) and a Shopping List Generator that will print out lists of ingredients automatically. By following the South Beach Diet Online, you'll not only get help gaining control of your weight and your heart health, you'll also be helping us make the diet better. Science is changing and improving all the time, and I see this diet as an evolution. As we learn new information about dieters' needs and experiences, we'll be able to continually improve the website, the plan and our ability to help people. To learn about changes and updates to the diet without registering for this site, visit *www.southbeachdiet.com/updates*

Dr Arthur Agatston